the
LOW CARBOHYD
diet

the LOW CARBOHYDRATE diet

Edited by Evelyn L. Fiore

MICHAEL JOSEPH – LONDON

First published in
Great Britain by
Michael Joseph Ltd
26 Bloomsbury Street
London W.C.1
November 1965
Second impression July 1966
Third impression September 1968
Fourth impression May 1969

Printed and bound
in Great Britain by
Richard Clay
(The Chaucer Press) Ltd
Bungay Suffolk

7181 0233 9

CONTENTS

*The editors are grateful
to Dr. Herman B. Zurrow of New York City
for much helpful comment and criticism supplied
while this manuscript was in preparation*

CHAPTER ONE

THE DIET THAT SPREAD UNDERGROUND

Some months ago in America, chronic weight-watchers became aware of a strange stirring in the world of nutrition . . . rumours of a diet which was achieving exciting results for people who had never before managed to get their weight problem under control.

Perhaps because it was habitually referred to as the 'Air Force' diet, without any official air force sanction, the new formula spread in a curiously underground fashion. It is now legend that copies of the diet were passed from friend to friend and run off on office Mimeograph machines. From the knowledgeable communications media, bits and pieces of material trickled down through the well-defined echelons of the 'in' groups—advertising, publishing, finance, and so on—until even in some of the better Seventh Avenue dress houses there were those who possessed perhaps a page of it and were thinking about trying it without exactly knowing what it was.

Then it began to surface. *Vogue* and *Redbook* brought it, in brief form, to public attention. A pamphlet entitled *The Drinking Man's Diet* carried its revolutionary message across the country, climaxing with a *Newsweek* report in which the word was blazoned wide that on this diet you can continue to drink. To dieters, this is indeed news; no other weight-watching diet puts up with liquor, with its enormous number of calories per drink.

But alcohol is not the only hitherto forbidden item which this new diet sanctions. Cream, butter, fried foods are allowed—heresy to those who know (and what dieter does not?) how many calories they contain. It became apparent that if this exceedingly valuable, exceedingly successful new approach to weight control were not to be misunderstood, it had better come out in full, understandable form with the background for its revolutionary approach made clear. Here, then, it is: the low carbohydrate diet works by cutting not *calories*, but *carbohydrates*. The principle, highly simplified, is that when fuel-producing carbohydrates are restricted, the body, which must burn something for energy, burns fat instead. It works so well that while the dieter is painlessly lowering his weight he has no trouble maintaining good health and high spirits.

FACING THE WORLD ON MELBA TOAST

The last consideration is important. If you are reading this book, you probably have dieted. You know what it means to face the world after breakfasting on dry Melba toast and a cup of black coffee. And you know how difficult it is to get through a morning's work when all you can think of is the delights that await you at lunchtime: a single breadstick partnered by a mound of grainy cottage cheese.

This state of demoralization, sometimes accompanied by nerve tantrums, is a familiar one to many a weight-watcher for a simple reason: whether he counts calories or puts himself on one of the fad 'crash' diets (all eggs, all bananas, all grapes or whatever), he takes off weight by cutting down on food. Now, any 'diet' will reduce you, in a manner of speaking, if it sharply reduces your food intake over a long enough period. Overweight is no problem in starving communities. This kind of diet will also reduce your vitality, your ability to function both physically and mentally, and even your life span if carried to foolish enough extremes.

THE BRINKMANSHIP SCHOOL OF DIETING

Low calorie diets, of course, are not starvation; they are brinkmanship. They offer the body just enough energy units to get along on, with none left over for storage or padding, and they will *generally* work *moderately* well for *some* people. The emphasis is intentional. For years the principle of calorie-cutting has been the ruling one in weight-watching circles, both medical and lay. Yet it has always been known that there are many for whom this principle will not work. For a great many others it can be made to work only by reducing their food intake to such pitiable proportions that nerves, personality, and productivity suffer. In extreme cases, the body itself can be so deprived of necessary nutrients that the slimming individual finds himself—or more probably herself—barely able to totter to the doctor's office so that restorative measures can be taken.

ALL THAT DIETING—AND NO RESULTS

Clearly, a healthy person of ordinary common sense will not choose to deplete his vitality, lower his resistance to infection, and court anaemia among other complex ailments merely in order to face himself more cheerfully in a full-length mirror. Well, there are serious reasons to worry about overweight. Its health hazards—some of which are discussed in Chapter Two—are well enough known to cause that same sensible person to take thought when his scale starts inching upward.

But—you're overweight. You have taken thought. You've tried starving, calorie-counting, exercise. In each case the results were the same—either there were none, or a few pounds slipped off only to be immediately replaced the moment you returned to anything like a normal diet. In addition you almost lost both your job and your marriage as it became impossible for any individual, however well adjusted, to get along with you. Yet still you waken to each new day aware that for another twenty-four hours you are going to ask your heart to service a plant that may be five, ten, or with really bad luck even twenty pounds heavier than it is efficiently equipped to manage. What to do?

First, if you haven't already done so, check with your doctor. Second (and contingent upon the outcome of that interview) read the rest of this book. The low carbohydrate diet may be your answer.

Suppose that you are fortunate enough to have a doctor whose concern for your health outweighs his verbal tact. He gives you a thoughtful look, puts down his pen and says, 'My friend, we are speaking not of overweight, but of obesity.'

In that case, forget this book, or give it to a friend. Obesity—gross overweight—is a medical classification, not a cosmetic one. If you are truly obese, neither this diet nor any other should be self-applied. You belong entirely in your doctor's hands, a slave to the letter of any regimen which he, after careful tests, tailors for *you*. It is possible that you are one of those individuals whose bodies, for reasons not yet fully understood, do not deal in the normal way with food.

The oldest clichés in the folklore of dieting are type A, who cannot look at a slice of beef without gaining four pounds, and type B, who remains underweight on a steady intake of heavy cream, French toast, and chocolate cake. The next time you overhear a luncheon conversation in which these two unfortunates are exchanging complaints, don't assume that A has been sneaking down to midnight feasts of fried pork chops and sweet potatoes, or that B is merely trying to endow herself with a touch of the piquantly peculiar. It is entirely possible that they are telling the truth. Any doctor numbers among his patients some who accumulate weight on very reasonable diets, and others who cannot cover their bones no matter how hard they try. The answer may be metabolic, psychological, glandular, or a complex combination of some or all of these; it may lie along biochemical lines yet to be explored. The one certainty is that in individuals at these extremes, body chemistry does not perform in the predictable manner.

'WE'LL CERTAINLY HAVE TO GET A FEW POUNDS OFF!'

But these, as we say, are extremes. Let us replay your scene with the doctor, who says cheerfully, 'Well, we'll certainly have to get a few pounds off you, won't we!' as he hoists you aboard his scales. In other words, you are overweight, not obese. If your excess weight is not the result of a metabolic or glandular disturbance, and if the doctor checks you out for any other health hazard which he feels might make a lowered carbohydrate regimen inadvisable for your particular system, then you're cleared to go on to Point Two.

At this point a few words of caution. This diet is designed for healthy people. Needless to say, if you are diabetic, anaemic, hypertense, or know yourself to be suffering from any other chronic disturbance, you will not undertake this or any other diet or alter your food habits in any way from the routine your doctor has prescribed. But even if you are in good health, *do not bypass the medical checkup*. No change in your way of life, particularly if you have not had a recent examination or are no longer as close to twenty-one as you once were, should be undertaken without a thorough physical going-over.

In view of the fact that cholesterol has become a household word during the past few years, the possible dangers of diet which does not restrict fat may occur to you even before you see your doctor. Discuss this with him. In all likelihood he will enlighten you on the current medical thinking along these lines, which is that while cholesterol may be involved in some way with arteriosclerosis and heart disease, it is no longer held to be the main factor. Too many aspects of the relationship between cholesterol and disease are still unexplored. A recent survey of cholesterol findings in geriatric cases involving arteriosclerosis showed a significant number of patients to have normal or low (depending upon the 'normal' standard accepted) cholesterol. There is, further, the fact that the body manufactures its own cholesterol, a certain amount of which is always present; despite the enormous flood of publicity which has succeeded in making cholesterol a fear symbol to the public, it has by no means been proven how diet affects the amount of cholesterol in the body, or how much. Let your doctor tell you whether or not the cholesterol controversy need have any bearing on your particular diet.

PROPORTION, NOT ELIMINATION

Another word you may want to bring up is ketosis. Perhaps your doctor will anticipate the question. Ketosis is a condition in which chemical compounds called ketones accumulate in the blood as a result of the incomplete oxidation of fat. An excess of ketone bodies can be harmful, even poisonous. In relation to the low carbohydrate diet, this has significance because it is generally accepted that fat cannot be completely broken down in the body unless carbohydrates are present. That is why, in the chapter discussing the application of the diet, we emphasize proportion, not elimination. You do not cut carbohydrates completely out of your food intake. You reduce them to 60 grams per day, unless your doctor approves a lower figure. You must continue to take in some carbohydrate—a measured quantity—in order to stay healthy.

A further caution: to repeat, this diet *works*. It has melted up to fourteen pounds a month off people who have never before managed to take off anything like that, stay healthy, and keep it off. But face this honestly: nothing will work if you gorge yourself. Further along, we give you *carte blanche* to eat as much as you like of certain foods. This is based on the assumption that you will like, or want, a more or less reasonable amount for your height, build, and way of life. If you are planning to use this diet as your Open Sesame to gross overeating, we must point out that while this diet has achieved startling, dramatic results, it has not—so far as we know—performed magic. If you are a neurotically compulsive overeater, you probably will be just as fat at the end of your diet as you are now, and you will have wasted a lot of time during which you should have been seeing a psychiatrist.

SELF-CONTROL EQUALS POUNDS OFF

On the other hand, if you are capable of a normal degree of self-control, you can launch yourself on the low carbohydrate diet with every assurance that pounds will start leaving you almost at once—often by the end of the second day. This alone is enough to boost the morale of the veteran dieter who has known the long agony of sweating out other diets—the weeks of waiting for the scales to prove what a good, self-denying boy (or girl) he has been.

But there are other advantages to this diet which no approach to the problem has ever before offered. Look (at the back of the book) at the meals you can eat! Observe that if you have been fighting for status as a fledgling gourmet, this diet in no way keeps you out of the club. You will find that the simple steak, crisply browned outside and rosy within, oozing delectable no-carbohydrate juices, is ideal for your purposes, but by no means all you are entitled to. You, or whoever cooks for you, can go high cuisine with wines, with herbs, with spices. With butter and *cream*. Malnourished reader, refugee from a thousand and one nights of sleepless fantasy about real food—on this diet you can have it.

And as for drinking, it's all true—on this diet you *can* drink. You can drink anything but beer, really sweet wines, or heavy liqueurs. It may cost a little more, or you may learn to drink a little less, but if you are ready to cooperate in these slight modifications, then the world of the convivial is still wide open to you. Crème de cacao-type ladies are perhaps the only ones who may be in for a real struggle as they try to make do with an after-dinner brandy instead of the vastly richer brew of their pre-diet choice.

Now, let's see how it works, and why.

CHAPTER TWO

THE HISTORY OF THE LOW CARBOHYDRATE DIET

The low carbohydrate diet represents a revolutionary principle of weight control in the sense that anything which attacks an entrenched regime is revolutionary. And the rule of the calorie count, in modern dietetic thinking, is certainly entrenched. So much so, that the most difficult thing you must do in order to benefit from the low carbohydrate diet is to put yourself through a certain amount of mental readjustment before you even begin to adjust your menu.

To borrow a concept from George Orwell, you will be required to do some nutritional Newthink. Dethrone the calorie. A considerable amount of research now indicates that it is not the number of calories you take in, but the kind, that affects the formation of body fat. You may be eating not too many calories, but more carbohydrate calories than your body can burn up.

Paradoxically, we can go back a hundred years and find an instance when this 'new' principle was put into successful operation. The results were spectacular then, but the basis for them was, by our present scientific evaluations, incompletely analysed and misunderstood. In consequence, the principle was sidetracked out of the mainstream of weight-control experimentation, and the calorie became king—or tyrant.

The episode was recorded for us by an otherwise uneminent Victorian, one William Banting. If you are addicted to the reading of Victorian novels, his name may ring a bell; somewhere you will have encountered young ladies who couldn't have a second bun for tea because they were 'banting'. Your eye may have slid over this as merely another example of that odd way the British have with slang: if the girl couldn't have seconds, she was obviously dieting, and what had 'banting' to do with dieting?

Had you been around at the time, you would have known. William Banting was a prosperous London coffin-maker who constructed final resting places for many notables of his time, the Duke of Wellington among them. It seems probable that Mr. Banting's apprentices did the actual woodwork involved, for his measurements make it difficult to see how he could have approached close enough to a workbench to be of much use. He stood less than five and a half feet tall and weighed something around fifteen stone. In his *Letter on Corpulence*, which he wrote in 1864 to acquaint the public with his dramatic and almost miraculous story, he makes the touching observation that he could not tie his own shoelaces or come down a flight of steps facing front. We can infer that he must have had trouble leading any kind of normal life.

DIETS THAT DIDN'T WORK

Mr. Banting was not happy with this state of affairs. He struggled for years to take off weight. He tried everything that the medical profession of that day would either sanction or not positively prohibit. He tried steaming, spas, starvation diets; he subjected himself to leeching and purging; he tried exercise, which must have taken superhuman effort in a man of his proportions. In 1862 William Banting was a discouraged—and still enormously heavy—gentleman in his sixties, who knew a great deal about the prevailing ideas in weight reduction—and knew that none worked for him.

Then Banting had an earache and realized that he was beginning to go deaf in one ear. For this reason, and no other, he consulted William Harvey, a noted ear, nose, and throat surgeon—a historic meeting in the annals of weight-control history. Harvey had recently returned from Paris, where he had heard the renowned French physiologist Claude Bernard describe some new theories about the role of the liver in body chemistry. Bernard believed that the liver secreted not only bile, but a sugar-like substance which it prepared at the expense of the blood elements that passed through it.

This theory had a profound effect on the study of diabetes. Harvey, who was much interested in diabetes, began to do a great deal of independent and evidently rather brilliant thinking on the whole question of how the body handles food elements, particularly fats, sugars, and starches. When William Banting presented himself, Harvey was as much interested in his obesity as he was in his ear, especially as the doctor soon satisfied himself that there was no organic reason for the ear trouble. Was it possible, Harvey wondered, that excess fat was pressing on some part of the inner ear, causing the pain and partial deafness?

A STARTLING EXPERIMENT

Nobody could have been readier than Banting to blame overweight for anything that went wrong with him. He became Harvey's willing, and shortly enthusiastic, collaborator in an experimental diet which was startling enough even for those days, when heavy eating was the fashion. It is truly shocking to today's weight-watchers, most of whom are so well schooled in computing calories that they can give you to the nearest fraction the caloric count of a dish containing fourteen ingredients from Upper Nepal.

For each meal, including breakfast, Banting was allowed up to 5 ounces of beef, mutton, kidneys, fish, bacon, venison, or any kind of poultry. (Today's average serving is 3–4 ounces.) He was to avoid sweets, flour, and starchy materials, but there were no similar restrictions as to the fat that came with his meat, so far as we know. He was permitted 3 or 4 ounces of biscuit, rusk, or toast; any vegetable except potato; as much tea as he liked without milk or sugar; a few ounces of fruit; and with lunch and supper two or three glasses of claret, sherry, or Madeira to wash down this considerable amount of food. He was permitted a nightcap of anything except champagne, port, or beer.

By modern calculation, William Banting must have been taking in not much less than 2800 calories a day. And in four months he had lost more than 20 lb. By the end of his first year on Harvey's diet he was 50 lb. lighter. His earache was long gone, his hearing restored. He was firmer and more vigorous than he had been in years. He had achieved this while eating fully and well, to say the least. He had been deprived only of sugars and starches. In other words, he had reduced dramatically, and without the slightest risk to his health, by practically eliminating carbohydrates from his daily food intake.

Understandably enthusiastic, Banting—who must have been a remarkable man—set to work to proselytize for this unorthodox, yet magnificently successful, treatment. At his own expense he published, in 1864, his now famous *Letter on Corpulence*. In it he described his diet, and added a heartfelt testimonial in which he tried to explain what it meant to a man of his history to be able to move about freely, exercise if he liked, and dress himself without assistance.

Banting's sincerity and his spectacular results impressed the public. But the medical profession was outraged, as he had suspected it would be, at the revolutionary suggestion that it might be possible to eat fat, among other things, to take fat off. The notion that a man might eat as much as he liked, as long as he excluded sugar and starch from his diet, was extraordinary enough. But that it should be put forward by a presumptuous layman without a scientific qualification to his name—Banting, in fact, gave the fullest possible credit to William Harvey, but this did not in the end do either of them much good—was more than the medical 'establishment' was prepared to put up with. It was pointed out with scorn that the material had not even appeared in any respectable professional organ. The whole idea was denounced as impertinent, ridiculous, dangerous.

RIDICULOUS? IT WORKS!

But meanwhile, many determined, or perhaps desperate, fat people tried Banting's diet, and found that ridiculous or not, it worked. This meant that the theory behind it could not be dismissed quite so lightly. The noted Dr. Felix von Niemeyer of Stuttgart undertook to investigate it, and succeeded in bringing off a curious shift of emphasis by which it was to appear that the meat in Banting's diet had been lean meat, trimmed of fat. He was left, therefore, with what we would now call a high protein diet, low in fat and carbohydrates. Dr. von Niemeyer was willing to go along with this, and with his endorsement so was every other physician interested in obesity.

These altered 'Banting Diets' became very popular, and explain how it was that 'banting' became synonymous with 'slimming' in England around the turn of the century. But to the end of his days William Banting maintained that the modified diet was, in principle and in practice, far inferior to the diet which had so altered his life and on which he had been allowed to eat plenty of fat with his meat.

Interesting confirmation that it was possible to get along with few or even no carbohydrates in the diet came in 1906, when a young Harvard anthropology instructor named Viljalmur Stefansson eagerly accepted a chance to go to the Arctic with the Leffingwell–Mikkelson Expedition. Stefansson—who afterwards of course became a world-famous anthropologist–explorer—went on ahead, planning to rendezvous with the expedition's ship at Herschel Island. But by some chance the rendezvous miscarried, and Stefansson was left to spend an Arctic winter with the Eskimos.

ARCTIC DIET: FISH WASHED DOWN WITH WATER

This was a rich research plum for a young scientist to chew on, but after a few days Stefansson began to fear that he might not live long enough to take advantage of it. His charming, cheerful, and hospitable hosts lived entirely on a diet of fish, washed down with water in which the gobbets of fish were briefly stewed. Stefansson's twentieth-century stomach rebelled at this primitive fare. He tried to improve it by broiling the fish, but this swiftly resulted in weakness, dizziness, and symptoms of malnutrition, and he deduced that on this highly restricted diet the body had to have not only the protein in the fish but the fat and other nutrient materials that were leached out into the water. Thus presented with a life-and-death reason for forcing down both fish and broth, Stefansson tried harder. Eventually he adjusted both physically and psychologically, and at the end of his time with the Eskimos, he had managed as well as any of them. In addition he felt fine and seemed in excellent condition.

He had also become exceedingly interested in the possibility that a diet high in proteins and fats and low in carbohydrates might serve all men better than the civilized diet of the world from which he had come. 'Balanced' meals in which relatively small amounts of meat or other protein were garlanded with rice, potatoes, or other starches, accompanied by bread and high-carbohydrate vegetables, followed by sweet desserts and sugared coffee . . . were these perhaps balanced in the wrong direction?

Like Banting, Stefansson began to hammer at the fortress of established nutritional thinking. He had about the same success. As the years went by his stature as anthropologist–explorer became enormous and unassailable, but his ideas about nutrition were simply bypassed.

Some time after his first experience with the Eskimo diet, Stefansson and a companion were sent to the Arctic by the American Museum of Natural History for a year of research. They were handsomely equipped with every necessity, including full stores for the year of 'civilized' food. But Stefansson and his companion, Dr. Anderson, elected to live in a fashion indigenous to the land they were studying. This meant a 'hunter's diet'—the fish they could catch, the meat they could kill, the water they could find—a way of life by which men had nourished themselves in the ages before they learned to plant and reap. The one-year project stretched into four, during which the two young men ranged over the Canadian Arctic, living entirely on their primitive diet. They found that when any component of it became scarce—as during one period when they had difficulty obtaining seal oil and had to eat lean caribou meat without additional fat—they became ill. As soon as the oil was restored, they recovered. As in Stefansson's earlier experience, he suffered no ill effects whatsoever, nor did Anderson, on what most nutritionists and certainly the ordinary civilized man would have considered a deprivation diet.

It seemed evident to Stefansson, as it had to Banting, that once adjusted to a plentiful diet in which only carbohydrates were restricted, his body would manufacture all the nutrients it needed for perfect functioning. He tested his theories later in controlled experiments, but although research along these lines was certainly being conducted at numerous nutritional study centres, nobody was ready to come forward with a positive statement that it was possible to stay healthy—perhaps healthier than you had ever been—to reduce excess fat, and to remain slender, muscular, and vigorous on a diet that ignored the total number of calories you ingested and concentrated instead on the amount of carbohydrate.

In 1928, Stefansson took part in a strictly controlled project at Bellevue Hospital, in which medical, nutritional, and anthropological experts from some of the most august institutions in the country hoped to learn more about what happened to the human body on an all-meat, non-vegetable, non-farinaceous diet. Research was directed by Dr. Eugene F. DuBois, medical director of the Russell Sage Foundation (subsequently chief physician at New York Hospital and Professor of Physiology at Cornell University Medical College). Once again Stefansson discovered that he could get along superbly on a combination of meats and fats, and that when fats were restricted he suffered. The absence of carbohydrate appeared to have only good effects. At the end of a year on this regimen, the research team reported that almost at once Stefansson had reduced a few pounds to his best normal weight, which he had thereafter maintained with no trouble. He showed no deficiency symptoms. His body appeared to have manufactured all its mineral and vitamin needs from the food it had been given. There was no loss of energy; in fact, as before, Stefansson functioned better than ever on this restricted diet and it seemed evident that when carbohydrate calories were not available for energy his body was perfectly capable of deriving what it needed from protein with fat.

The results of the test were of course published, but they left the general public cold. People were convinced that a diet which offered you as much meat as you could eat (the research indicated that a person on this diet would be able to eat, and would have appetite for, only as much as his body required) and which included the dreaded item *fat*, could result only in supplying a lethal number of calories. The possibility that it was not the number but the kind, and how the body used them, that added up to excess fat, simply had no appeal.

CALORIES: THE BEGINNING OF THE END

Science, however, was interested. In 1944 Dr. Blake F. Donaldson conducted a famous experiment with obese patients at New York Hospital, reducing them on diets high in proteins and fats. Dr. Donaldson's book, *Strong Medicine*, was another signpost along the road on which Banting had embarked eighty years earlier. But the average dieter went on counting calories, all kinds together, oblivious that more and more research was piling up to suggest that with his low calorie carrot salad, high in carbohydrates, he was doing his measurements more harm than if he had satisfied his hunger with a nice slice of ham—higher in total calories, but zero in carbohydrates.

A few years afterwards the E.I. du Pont company headquarters in Wilmington, Delaware, undertook a weight-control programme involving a group of its executives who had been unsuccessful with low calorie diets. Under the direction of Dr. Albert W. Pennington and Dr. George H. Gehrmann, director of du Pont's medical division, these overweight individuals were allowed all the protein and fat they wanted. Total caloric intake was unrestricted, in some cases going up to 3000 or more calories per day—but carbohydrate was withheld. The results were spectacular. The weight losses varied from person to person, as did the time required for each to reach his goal. But, averaged out, each dieter lost 22 lb. in slightly more than three months.

This time public imagination was captured. *Holiday* magazine ran a series of articles discussing the du Pont project, and for a time the so-called Holiday Diet became a household word. In principle, this was a controlled-carbohydrate diet, but in practice the high-protein, high-fat regimen offered so many calories per day that it was still impossible for most people to believe it would work. The medical directors of the project knew, and had proved, that when carbohydrate was not present the body would burn fat instead.

However, in the years that followed, so much significant research has been recorded by so many authoritative investigators that it is no longer possible to dismiss the low carbohydrate diet as interesting but freakish. At Middlesex Hospital in London, a team headed by Professor Alan Kekwick and biochemist Dr. G. L. S. Pawan undertook an intensive study of diet involving both obese and non-obese subjects, the results of which have had enormous impact on weight-control theory. They found that obese patients would lose weight even on comparatively high calorie diets so long as the calories consisted chiefly of protein and fat, and the carbohydrates were kept to a minimum. They also concluded that on a fat and protein diet, low in carbohydrate, the body would derive its nutritional requirements from the food which it was given.

This is a skimming of the research bloodlines behind the low carbohydrate diet. The serious student with time to invest and the desire to know more can find a mountain of relevant material at his nearest library. The serious dieter needs only to start cutting carbohydrates; he will lose weight.

CHAPTER THREE

HOW THIS DIET WORKS—AND WHY

From our school days on, we have all been made thoroughly familiar with certain basic facts about food. It is that which can be taken into the body, digested, and used for growth, repair, and energy. Most of us can close our eyes and see, tacked up on the classroom wall, that familiar, many-coloured chart which was designed to imprint on our memories the 'Basic Seven', the nutritional categories from which our daily food supply must be composed if we were to grow up strong, straight-spined, and brainy . . . leafy green and yellow vegetables, citrus fruits, other fruits and vegetables, milk and its products, the meat group, breads and cereals, butter or fortified margarine.

On this diet (with extras like an occasional chocolate bar or a dry Martini) most Americans do manage very well. They grow taller than their forefathers, live longer, and have consistently produced athletes who commanded front-rank places in the international picture. Only recently have American athletes had to struggle for pre-eminence as other nations, benefiting from diets and living standards improved since the Second World War, have begun to offer powerful challenges.

But some people—as you know because you are reading this book—do not manage quite so well. They get fat.

Sometimes, of course, this happens because the occasional chocolate bar has snowballed into an addiction to sweets and pastries. Sometimes it can be traced to simple overeating of everything in sight; sometimes to a 'need' to relax with five beers a night and all the pretzels you can get hold of. Sometimes, however, an individual accumulates fat on a reasonably balanced diet on which he can prove to his doctor and to his own conscience that he has not overindulged.

Overweight, of course—unless it amounts to obesity, about which there can be no two opinions—can be a somewhat elastic concept. William Banting was certainly obese, and even in his day, before the succeeding years of research which established the connection between obesity and certain diseases, both he and his doctor knew something had to be done about it. But if he had been merely a portly man, of well-fed appearance, he would have been considered exceedingly odd to be disturbed about his weight. A noted politician of that day was widely quoted as having declared that he never could put his trust in a man who didn't have to lean backward just a bit to support his own weight. Indeed, until around the time of the First World War, the popular concept of a truly solid citizen decreed that his waistline must reflect his bank account—both must be substantial. Slenderness in youth was acceptable, but as a man grew older it was expected that both he and his family would display, in their measurements, how well he was able to feed them.

Other times, other ways. A glance at the weight chart included at the back of this book will indicate what very different standards we hold today about desirable, healthful weight. As a matter of fact, most women will confess, to everyone except their doctors, that they consider even these widely accepted weight allowances to be excessive. 'If I weighed that much I'd be a mountain!' many a five-foot-two lady has been heard to exclaim upon checking the 'normal' weight range for her size—somewhere between 7 st. 12 lb. and 8 st. 13 lb. Possibly she has not taken her build into consideration, possibly her age. But possibly she is right. The life-insurance companies which compile most of these tables know that year by year the desirable-weight range tends to come down.

But, of course, the modern estimate of what constitutes overweight and how important it is to control it, is not influenced solely by the desire to possess a slender, well-knit body that can show off one's clothes to the greatest advantage. Expanding research and an increasing weight of statistical evidence have alerted us to the relationship between excess weight and good health and life expectancy. If you are over thirty-five and have shown a recent tendency to expand more than a bit, your doctor has already reminded you that every pound you put on increases your vulnerability to hypertension, diabetes, arthritis, and a frightening list of cardiovascular and kidney diseases. Nor are the surgeons overly cheerful when an overweight patient requires an operation, for even relatively common procedures, like hernia corrections and appendectomies, can be complicated by layers of excess fat. Further, corpulent patients require a much longer convalescence, not only from surgery but from illness as well.

Insurance tables also supply the portmanteau statistic in which all the other risks are summed up: after 45, with every 10 lb. of excess weight you put on you increase by roughly 10 per cent your chances of early death.

We will take it, therefore, as read that you have a weight problem and that for social, sartorial, and health reasons, as well as a dozen other reasons best known to yourself, you are determined to solve it by going on a diet.

For many years the standard approach to correction has been to start watching calories. Accepted by doctor and layman alike has been the dictum that if you put on weight it was because you were feeding your body more calories than it required for a day of normal operation. It frugally deposited the oversupply in the liver and in other tissues, to be drawn on as needed. But if the oversupply continued to be too lavish, or if not enough of it was needed—in other words if you consistently overate and did not take enough exercise—you were in trouble.

'CALORIE'—A DIRTY WORD?

If you will approach the calorie as though it were neither a trapped tiger, a dram of arsenic, nor a dirty word, you will doubtless remember that technically it is simply a measurement. Specifically, it is the amount of heat required to raise the temperature of 1 lb. of water 4 degrees F. Nutritionally, it refers to the units of heat, or energy, which the body gets from its food.

Years of research, of course, have standardized what science considers a desirable range of caloric intake for the average person. The daily amount recommended by nutritionists for a healthy adult woman in a moderately active way of life is 2500, for a man, 3000—adjusted to height and build. The caloric approach to weight reduction often requires a cutback to 1000 or 1200 calories a day. Clearly this cannot be accomplished without hardship.

For some dieters, the prize is worth the game. Embarking upon a low calorie diet, they find their weight coming down; they avoid nervous collapse, and with luck and exceeding care manage not to damage their vital functions. A sharp calorie cut, of course, cannot be sustained for more than a short period. Having lost a few pounds, the dieter gratefully returns—as his body signals that he must—to a fuller diet. What generally happens, as survivors of 'crash' diets know, is that in reaction to the days, or weeks, of near-starvation they start stuffing themselves with less control than ever. Before they know it the wheel comes full circle and they are once again looking for the newest, quickest way to shave off their reacquired adipose tissue.

Nevertheless, there are people who can reduce on low calorie diets without becoming caught in this cycle. By cutting down their over-all food intake by a sensible percentage they can get down to a good weight—and most adults know, by the way they feel and look, more or less to a pound what their best weight is—and stabilize there merely at the cost of maintaining a constant watchfulness over how much they eat. The low carbohydrate diet was not designed for those who have been truly successful with low calorie diets.

THE OLDER, THE LESS WEIGHT

What is significant about this 'new' approach—which has been shown to be far from a Johnny-come-lately into weight control theory—is that it will reduce those who have trimmed down their calories until they couldn't stand it any more, only to find that their waist-lines haven't trimmed down at all. For these people, carbohydrate control can be not merely a way of taking off a few pounds, but the foundation of a whole new philosophy of eating which may make it easy for them to maintain their own best weight, and a well-nourished body, for the rest of their lives.

Again, remember: in extreme cases the answer to overweight may be metabolic or glandular, and should be discovered and handled by your doctor. But if your metabolism registers within normal range, and no glandular imbalance shows up, current nutritional thinking offers you this hope: it is possible that your body does not utilize its food—specifically, its carbohydrates—in the 'normal' manner.

Food is accepted into the body as protein, fat, or carbohydrate. Protein, which derives its name from a Greek word meaning 'of first importance', is literally that—the fundamental nutrient without which no animal can survive. It is involved in the structure of every cell of the body. It builds and maintains body tissues, contributes to the formation of antibodies that resist infection, and performs other complex functions, some of which have only lately come under investigation. Protein varies in quality. We derive most of our prime protein supply from animal foods like meat, fish, poultry and eggs, and milk and milk products. Certain beans and nuts supply it, as to a lesser degree do vegetables. As more of the world opens up for study, there appears to be growing evidence that where protein is derived more from plants than from animals, people tend to be smaller than they are in places where good quality protein is plentiful. For example, Orientals, who must satisfy their food needs largely with grains and cereals, are, as a group, far smaller than Australians and New Zealanders, who consume a quantity of meat enormous even by American standards. Whatever other factors may be involved, it is certain that diet to some extent accounts for such physical differences.

THE SIGNIFICANCE OF THE NEW APPROACH

In terms of fuel, 1 gram of protein supplies 4 calories. (A gram equals about $\frac{1}{4}$ teaspoon.) But the biochemical processes by which the body breaks down protein for its various uses are so complex that the fuel value of the protein is not quickly available.

Fats supply vitamins and essential fatty acids which, so far as we presently know, the body cannot obtain from other substances. Fats are present in both plant and animal foods, but again the meat group (including milk products) supplies about 60 per cent to the vegetable group's 40 per cent. Like protein, fat digests slowly, which contributes to what is called its 'satiety value': when fat is present in your diet you tend to feel less hungry than you do on a fat-free regimen. Remember this if the high caloric count of fat starts you wondering all over again how you can possibly lose weight on a diet that allows you butter and cheese! One gram of fat supplies 9 calories—more than twice as much energy per unit than an equal weight of carbohydrates, which are popularly thought to be the body's chief source of fuel.

Now, the average person metabolizes his food efficiently. His body grows, keeps itself in good repair, burns what it requires for energy, and, as has been indicated, stores up the rest to be used as needed, some in the liver, and some as body fat. It is important to remember that fats *and* carbohydrates are stored in this way. (It is an interesting sidelight on the activity in nutritional research that until very recently science considered it established that protein was used or excreted by the body, and never stored. Current investigation, however, may show that certain forms of protein may be stored in some manner or quantity as yet unknown.) When our average person feels that he is 'storing' a bit too much, he cuts down his total food intake and the excess, very likely, comes off.

THE VALUE OF FAT

But what happens when a healthy body plant doesn't operate in this manner—when the restricted food intake is not followed by a loss of excess weight? What happens in the body to prevent it from responding in a predictable manner?

We must go back to Banting and Harvey, who first indicated by their successful experiment that carbohydrates might be to blame, and follow the line of research and experiment to its latest expression in the low carbohydrate diet to reach the answer. If you cannot lose weight by following orthodox nutritional patterns, you may be the victim of a fairly common biochemical quirk which keeps your body from burning up its carbohydrate intake at the normal rate, and stores it up instead as fat.

Because controlled-carbohydrate diets get the right results, we know that this happens. But precisely how it happens is not so easily demonstrated. One theory suggests that a hormone or enzyme deficiency may be to blame. Another, and a possibly related one, is concerned with the subtle interactions of body chemistry and metabolism far too complex for the layman really to follow. In every important research centre, physiologists, biochemists, and nutritionists are investigating these problems; for our purposes it is enough to know that carbohydrate control works in weight reduction.

If this smacks of the 'I don't know much about art but I know what I like' school of thought, reflect that the science of nutrition itself, as applied to actual food programmes, did not get under full sail much before the start of the twentieth century, when researchers established the importance of protein in the animal world. Man, of course, has been interested in the quantity, quality, and taste of his food ever since he has been around to eat it, but until recently his food habits reflected his standards of living, not his understanding of what happened to the food inside him, because this knowledge was not available. The poor and simple have always subsisted on whatever they could catch, kill, or grow most handily. The rich, as far back as pre-Biblical times, were wont to live on rich meats and 'the fat of the land'. In more sophisticated civilizations, the truly riotous liver expanded his horizons by combining flavours and adding spices to his viands. Through trial and error they all found out that there were things they could digest and things they couldn't. It has remained for the laboratories and research teams of this century to start telling us how, and why, this happens.

THE IMBALANCE OF THE BALANCED DIET

Like all other branches of science, nutrition has progressed at an intensified rate since the Second World War. New machines and methods—particularly the use of radioactive isotopes and 'tagging' so that the activities of given substances within the body can be actually traced—together with vastly increased armies of trained investigators, are building up an enormous amount of data never before available. The jet-age opportunity for swift access to hitherto little-known peoples and their alien ways of life has opened up new research roads. From the main highway of the 'Basic Seven', exploratory offshoots are being made, as we learn that people—like the Eskimos and like various tribes in Africa and remote sections of India—have maintained excellent health, physique, and morale on all-meat diets. (According to the Canadian ethnologist Jenness and to others who have lived among the Eskimos, their appearance of rotundity is due largely to their garments, not to a prevalence of excess fat.) And while the Grenfell Mission of 1892 found that scurvy, rickets, and other deficiency diseases were certainly not unknown among the Eskimos of Labrador, later investigations suggested that these problems followed upon the introduction to these groups of the white man's more agrarian diet.

Obviously these nutritional byways are not conclusive. But they suggest that continued investigation may one day throw new light on our present concept of the 'balanced' diet. In the meantime, it has been demonstrated that human beings can manage very well when the proportion of carbohydrate to fat and protein in their diet is taken far below hitherto accepted levels—and that for people who cannot control their overweight problem in other ways, carbohydrate control is the answer.

Carbohydrate *control*—not elimination. Weight-watchers who have become sensibly sceptical of extremist fads will observe that this diet is not an all-or-nothing crash programme. It offers *fewer* carbohydrates, not *no* carbohydrates. It offers you a full, satisfying diet. There is no danger of the total collapse of will that so often sends the low-calorie dieter on frantic refrigerator raids, because being well supplied with slowly digested fats and proteins, you never become that hungry. Further, it offers substantial amounts of food that are worth eating, with taste possibilities bounded only by the cook's time and/or talent. No diet has ever offered more—or as much.

SCEPTICS: NOW HEAR THIS

But perhaps most important to the chronic weight-watcher is that this diet works in two ways. It works not only to take weight off, but to keep it off. Once you have trained yourself to recognize high carbohydrate foods (and the only surprises here are in the areas of certain fruits and vegetables which we are not accustomed to thinking of in these terms), and to restrict them so that your diet delivers no more than 60 carbohydrate grams per day, you have adopted a painless, self-propelled eating pattern which will control your weight for good.

Try it. People will soon be saying to you what was said recently to a pretty teen-ager, a veteran of low-calorie diets which had offered only temporary results, by an envious friend: 'Gosh, Emily—this time you've retained your weight loss!'

CHAPTER FOUR

HOW YOU CAN BENEFIT BY THIS DIET

Having come this far, and having glanced at the recipes and menus that follow, you know that this diet will not call upon you for heroism above and beyond your strength of character. Once you have trained yourself to edit out the extra carbohydrates, your food allowance is so liberal and satisfying, and can be so interesting, that it can give rise to another sort of problem.

Recently a group of teachers in a suburban school decided to try the low carbohydrate diet together, so that they could draw on each other for moral and technical support and enliven their menus by exchange of recipes. By the end of the first week they had all lost between three and six pounds, and by the end of the third week most of them had put in happy hours taking in their skirts and shifts. But one young second-grade teacher continued to appear in her pre-diet wardrobe, unaltered, though her mirror must have told her that she looked baggier every day. Finally a colleague, who knew Miss X wasn't much of a hand with a sewing machine, made a tactful offer of help.

'It's not the sewing!' Miss X burst out. 'I've always had to pay for alterations and I don't mind that. I'm just afraid to believe it, that's all. I'm three inches less around the hips but I just *know* that the minute I get those skirts taken in those inches will be back. Nobody can take off weight this easily!'

Miss X was suffering from her American heritage of post-Puritan conscience: it can't be good for you unless it hurts.

Well, this diet is good for you, and it's good for your figure, and it will hurt less than any reducing regimen you've ever tried. You'll never go hungry. It is also very easy to apply because it's loaded with foods that have probably always formed the mainstay of your menu—meats, fish, poultry, eggs, cheese that you like to eat.

But if, like Miss X, you can't accept happiness without knowing that it's going to cost you something—relax. It will require some effort at first. If you are an old-line dieter, you probably do not realize how conditioned you are to the calorie-counting dogma. It takes a tricky bit of mental adjustment to stop thinking of calories as little horned men with pitchforks at the ready, just waiting for you to glance at Beef Stroganoff on a menu.

The best way to do it is to stop thinking about calories *altogether*. Think in terms of *grams*. The diet list is set up that way, as are the long food charts which have been appended to make it simple for you to keep your menu varied, yet still within your 60-gram limit. Food elements translate very easily from grams to calories. When you eat 1 gram of carbohydrate, remember, you're getting 4 calories; 1 gram of protein, 4; 1 gram of fat, 9. But don't translate. The reason for this is simple but crucial. This diet is carefully balanced to maintain a proportion of carbohydrate to protein and fat. It reduces carbohydrate, but supplies you with fat and protein to perform their own functions and also to fill in for the carbohydrate you've cut down. When you allow yourself to think in terms of calories—particularly of calories of fat—you tend to worry about how many you're taking in. Almost involuntarily you start holding back, cutting down on everything, trapped again by the calorie-counter's credo that if less is good, much less must be better. Shortly you are hungry, fretful, easily tired. You blame it on the diet, but the fault is yours because you have not played by the rules. You must have the protein to feed your muscles, bones, and tissues; you must have the fat for energy, for satiety, for keeping the body supple, for production of fatty acids.

FORGET THE TOTAL AMOUNT

Forget the total amount you are eating of the foods you are allowed. Concentrate only on the carbohydrate-loaded foods; they are the only ones you need to worry about.

So you see, though you may eat with sinful-seeming freedom, you will still be in a position to worry if worry you must.

You can also worry, in a very minor way, about drinking. Needless to say, if you have a Drinking Problem, you have more to worry about than your weight, and this book will not be of much help. But if you are only concerned with the odd glass, the ritual cocktail hour, or the big party, a glance at the Alcoholic Beverages Chart will cheer you. It has never before been known to cheer dieters, because 1 gram of alcohol contains 7 calories. But we said you could drink on this diet, and we meant it. As the table shows, the number of *carbohydrates* per average drink is comparatively low, with the exception of beer, ale, sweet wines, and liqueurs. This admits liquor, within reason and with the discretion which will naturally accompany the thinking man's drinking even if he is not overweight, to the low carbohydrate dieter's list of pleasures.

Why, then, do so many non-teetotallers put on weight? For one thing, they eat while they're drinking. They eat tasty bits of things spread on bread (12 grams carbohydrate per slice) and piled on tiny crackers (much lower, around 3 each, but they still add up by the handful). They eat delightful specialties-of-the-house which have been rolled in breadcrumbs (more than 8 grams per ounce). They eat potato crisps uncountable, which average 1 gram per crisp, and they frequently dip these into spreads which have been made with cornstarch or flour.

There is also the possibility, presently under investigation, that because alcohol is absorbed much more swiftly into the system than solid foods, its calories can be immediately utilized to supply some of the body's energy needs. By the time food calories are available fewer of them are required, and thus more are left over to settle down upon the waistlines of the unwary.

THE WISE CAN CONTINUE TO DRINK

But as the low carbohydrate dieter is not unwary, he or she may continue to drink so long as it is remembered that while 60 grams of carbohydrate per day are allowed, it would really be rather unwise to take them all in the form of liquor and tidbits. The joys of a nice slice of hot buttered toast with your breakfast egg are not to be belittled. Do you really want to give that up for twelve potato crisps?

Attitude and alcohol, then, are two items to think about as you incorporate the low carbohydrate diet into your way of life—and alcohol only because of what often goes with it. Beyond that, you can put yourself on this diet in the time it takes to memorize two simple rules. *Keep down* your intake of sugars and starches. *Keep up* your intake of fats and proteins. Remember: on this diet, you can eat all you want of the foods that are high in protein and fat as long as they are low in carbohydrate. Best of all to remember—*you need never be hungry.*

To follow the first rule, it will help to start out by ruling all these off your permitted list:

cakes, cupcakes
pies, puddings
all other desserts made with sugar and/or thickeners such as flour, cornstarch, etc.
all canned or stewed fruits cooked with sugar or syrup
all cereals and cereal products
all jams, jellies, candies, syrups, honey, sugar
all rice and pasta (spaghetti, macaroni, noodles)
all dried fruits
all biscuits and extra bread
lima beans, corn, peas, okra, potatoes
apples, apricots, bananas, orange juice, peaches, pears, plums, pineapple, watermelon; all berries except strawberries
all sweet carbonated drinks
all beer and sweet wines

Please note that this is *the way you start out.* You are not going to have to bear the rest of your years without ever tasting these foods again. The reason you outlaw them just at first is to train your eye and your habits—to learn so well that you know without having to stop and think just which foods deliver the highest number of carbohydrates.

THE ADVISABILITY OF VITAMIN SUPPLEMENTS

Meanwhile, your doctor may suggest a vitamin supplement to bolster your intake of vitamin C, the B-complex vitamins, or other nutrients. Check with him as to the advisability of such a supplement.

If you will check the comprehensive Food Values table, you will readily see that most of the foods which have not been prohibited—and that's most of them!—contain some carbohydrate. Many of the permitted fruits and vegetables contain a fair amount. Unless you stop eating, in the ordinary course of events you will be taking in a small amount of carbohydrate even with the high carbohydrate items nowhere around. Being allowed a total of 60 grams per day, you begin to juggle and balance.

As you grow adept at the balancing act, you can begin to sneak back into your diet small portions of the outlawed items. Bread, for instance, is the most difficult thing for most weight-watchers to give up. Notice on the preceding list that you have not been asked to give up all bread; only extra bread. What's extra? That depends on you. You don't have to punish yourself. By switching from orange to grapefruit juice, and cutting that down to 2 ounces instead of the usual 4, you can give yourself a breakfast of juice, two scrambled eggs, a slice of buttered toast, and coffee with cream and non-caloric sweetener (the type low in carbohydrate) without taking in more than 18 or so carbohydrate grams, depending on the size of the eggs and the thickness of the bread.

OFF TO A WELL-FILLED START

This sounds like a lot. But you've got your day off to a sound, well-filled start. Your morning is energetic, cheerful, your imagination constructively occupied with the creation of better money-making schemes instead of being bogged down on the subject of food. You can lunch on an average portion of shrimp—oven fried—plus six or seven stalks of asparagus vinaigrette, and add only 17 grams. This leaves you about 25 grams—if you want to be super-cautious, 20 grams—to play about with at dinner. No bread, plenty of meat, low carbohydrate vegetable or salad if you like, and even a small portion of mashed potato ($\frac{1}{4}$ cup, with butter and milk, will run you only about 6 grams) can be your happy lot, and if you finish off with a nice bit of cheese you might even—depending on the size of your portions of other food—allow yourself a saltine for it to sit upon. Your unsugared or artificially sweetened tea or coffee hardly counts. Starvation? Deprivation? Not by any standard. And as you can see, the juggling possibilities are limited only by your personal tastes. Give up the breakfast juice, confine yourself to one egg, leave the French dressing off your asparagus at lunchtime, and have an extra slice of bread if bread you must have. The beauty of this diet is that, while you must still juggle, at least you've got something to juggle.

As you begin to reinstate carbohydrate-significant foods to your diet, bear in mind the word *portions*. The comprehensive Food Values tables are calculated upon so-called 'average' portions. As you are allowed to eat more than enough to satisfy you of filling, high protein foods and fats, it involves small sacrifice to keep portions of other foods down to a bit less than average until you have determined at what rate your personal body chemistry can cope with carbohydrates and still keep off excess weight on a long-term, satisfactory basis.

CARBOHYDRATES ARE THE VILLAINS

In that last sentence lies concealed a secret message, and each dieter must work out its meaning for himself. Sixty grams of carbohydrate per day has been set as the maximum which the average individual can allow himself in order to achieve a satisfactory, steady weight reduction. It is here that you start out. As you go on, you may find that you are not losing weight fast enough to keep you happy. In that case, ask your doctor if you can trim down your carbohydrate intake to 50 grams a day, and try a short walk before breakfast. The chances are that if the diet is not working quickly enough to satisfy you, it is not because it is wrong for you, but because you haven't yet discovered the precise proportion of carbohydrate to protein and fat which will work best for you. Taking it down a few grams will usually do the trick—but keep in mind that the danger of ketosis makes it essential that you check with your doctor first.

On the other hand, there are those fortunate types who, having lost as much as they hoped to on 60 grams a day, find that they can start inching upward by minute steps until they are taking in perhaps 65 or even more grams a day, while still, like the teen-ager previously cited, retaining their weight loss. It is premature here to emphasize this, because you must start out with 60; but it is nice to know that though this diet is full, satisfying, and tasty, you may be one of the lucky ones who can eventually go on to even better things.

Meanwhile, start with 60. Make meat, fish, poultry, and eggs the backbone of your diet. Go cautiously in the direction of all desserts, all flour, potatoes, noodles, rich dishes, all addenda like honey and jam. Shun candy, sweet soft drinks, beer. You must snack between meals? A slice of cheese, a few almonds, an olive or two, dried crisp bacon curls (here is one cocktail-type tidbit you can dip into) should pacify your craving—but face facts, they do add something; you'll have to either trim the extra grams off something else or, better still, train yourself not to snack. It *can* be done.

In stews and gravies, experiment. Omit flour and cornstarch thickeners and rely instead on flavour-building spices, herbs, and wines to make these items more appealing than ever before. However, don't lose your head; if, in dining out, you cannot avoid a dish in which some thickener was used, try to eat as much of the solid portion and as little of the sauce as possible—and remember that if two or three tablespoons of flour were used to thicken a stew served to six people, your allotment of it is not really going to be disastrously large.

As a matter of fact, a cook's tour of favourite recipes will be a remarkably cheering experience for the low carbohydrate dieter. Barring desserts—and barring of course main-dish recipes based on noodles or pasta or other starch —so many of the meat, fish, and poultry recipes that you like can be adapted so easily to this diet that unless you prefer to live simply on plain foods you certainly don't have to. The menus and recipes included in this book have been organized to show what can be done; they are far from the limit of what you can do, if you have the time, taste, and mind to do it.

COMPARED TO CALORIE COUNTING, CHILD'S PLAY

On this diet you will eat fully and well. You will reduce quickly down to your own best weight and will at the same time form new eating patterns which will maintain this weight for you easily. You will accomplish this without endangering your health, disrupting your way of life, making yourself anathema to friends and co-workers, or creating soap-opera spectaculars about your sufferings (because there won't be any) unless you want to. You will avoid depression, low energy, and nervous strain induced by semi-starvation; if you have a nasty temper you will have to find some other excuse to explain it. You can enjoy your liquor like any other civilized human being.

What are you waiting for?

CARBOHYDRATE CONTENT OF COMMON FOODS

TABLE OF FOOD VALUES IN COMMON PORTIONS

[alphabetically]

Amounts of food on this table refer to edible portions only. All spoonful measurements are level. All cup and portion of cup measurements are scant unless otherwise cited. Fruit measurements include skin unless otherwise noted. Please note that caloric values, which have no significance in the low carbohydrate diet, have been included here purely as a point of interest and comparison for the curious.

Food	Amount	Carbo-hydrate (grams)	Cals.
Almonds	12–15	**5**	90
Angel Food Cake	2″ section	**24**	108
Apple, raw	1 small	**15**	58
frozen, sliced, sweetened	⅔ cup	**24**	92
Apple Juice	½ cup	**17**	47
Apple Pie	1 medium slice	**53**	331
Apple Sauce, sweetened	½ cup	**24**	72
unsweetened	½ cup	**12**	42
Apricots, raw	3 medium	**13**	51
canned, water	½ cup	**10**	38
canned, syrup	½ cup	**22**	86
dried, uncooked	5 medium halves	**13**	52
cooked, sweetened	½ cup	**31**	183
frozen	½ cup	**25**	98
Artichokes			
Globe, boiled	1 medium	**5·5**	8
Jerusalem, boiled	1 oz.	**9·0**	5
Asparagus, cooked, fresh, or frozen	6–7 spears	**4**	20
canned, drained	6–7 spears	**3**	21
Avocados	half, peeled	**6**	167

Food	Amount	Carbo-hydrate (grams)	Cals.
Bacon	2 strips	Tr.	97
Bananas	1 small	22	85
Bean Sprouts	½ cup	3	17·5
Beef, various cuts, braised, pot-roasted, lean, and fat	3½ oz.	0	288
Beef Bouillon Soup	1 cup	2·5	32
Beef Liver, fried	3½ oz.	5	229
Beef Stew (with veg.)	½ cup	7	107
Beetroot, cooked or canned, drained	½ cup	9	35
Blackberries, raw	½ cup	9	40
canned, water	½ cup	9	43
canned, syrup	½ cup	22	91
Blueberries, raw	⅔ cup	15	61
frozen, no sugar	⅔ cup	14	56
canned, water	½ cup	10	37
canned, syrup	½ cup	26	98
Blueberry Pie	1 medium slice	51	291
Blue Cheese	1 oz.	1	104
Bologna Sausage	3½ oz.	7	300
Bouillon Cubes	1	Tr.	2
Brains, calves', boiled	3½ oz.	1	102
Brazil Nuts	⅔ cup	11	654
Bread Crumbs	1 cup	72	385
Broccoli, cooked	⅔ cup	5	26
Brown Bread	1 small slice	23	105
Brown Sugar	1 tbs.	13	48
Brussels Sprouts	¾ cup	7	36
Butter	1 tbs.	Tr.	100
Buttermilk	½ cup	5	36
Butterscotch	3½ oz.	86	410
Cabbage, raw	Section app. 3″ × 4″	5	24
cooked	1⅔ cup	4	20
Calves' Liver, fried	3½ oz.	4	261
Camembert Cheese	1 oz.	1	85
Cantaloupe	½ cantaloupe	8	30
Caramels	3½ oz.	78	415

Food	Amount	Carbo-hydrate (grams)	Cals.
Carrots, raw	1 medium or ½ cup grated	4·5	21
cooked, drained	½ cup	5	22
canned, drained	½ cup	5	22
Cashew Nuts	¼ cup	9	168
Cauliflower, raw	½ cup	3	15
cooked, drained	½ cup	3	15
Celery, raw	½ cup diced	2	12
Celery Soup, creamed	1 cup	17·5	162
Cheddar Cheese	1 oz.	1	113
Cheddar Cheese, processed	1 oz.	1	105
Cherries, raw	½ cup	8	32
canned, sour red	½ cup	15	60
Cherry Pie	1 medium slice	55	340
Chicken, broiled	3½ oz.	0	218
Chicken Liver, cooked	3½ oz.	3	165
Chicken Noodle Soup	1 cup	7·5	65
Chicken Soup, creamed	1 cup	15	182
Chilli Sauce	1 tbs.	4	17
Chocolate, bitter	1 oz.	8	142
bittersweet	1 oz.	14	143
Chocolate, milk	1 oz.	16	143
Chocolate, milk with almonds	1 oz.	14	151
Chocolate Milk	1 cup	22	148
Chocolate Syrup	1 tbs.	13	49
Chopped Beef, creamed	3½ oz.	7	154
Clam Chowder	1 cup	12·5	82
Clams, canned, undrained	3½ oz.	3	51
Cocoa	1 cup	27	236
Coconut, fresh, shredded	½ cup	4·5	173
dried, shredded	½ cup	16·5	173
Cod, broiled	3½ oz.	0	170
dried	3½ oz.	0	375
Condensed Milk, canned	½ cup	84	490
Corn, fresh, cooked	1 small ear	18	91
canned, cream style	½ cup	20	82
canned, whole kernel	½ cup	16	66
Corned Beef, canned	3½ oz.	0	212

Food	Amount	Carbo-hydrate (grams)	Cals.
Corned Beef Hash, canned	3½ oz.	**7**	140
Corn Flakes	1 cup	**21**	95
Cornmeal, all kinds	½ cup	**11**	50
Cornstarch	1 tbs.	**7**	29
Cottage Cheese, uncreamed	1 oz.	**1**	26
Crab, hard shell	3½ oz.	**1**	101
Crabs, canned or cooked	3½ oz.	**1**	101
Crackers			
saltine	2 whole	**6**	34
soda	1 medium	**4**	22
Cranberries, raw	½ cup	**6**	23
canned, strained	½ cup	**38**	46
Cream, light	1 tbs.	**1**	31
heavy	1 tbs.	**Tr.**	53
sour	1 tbs.	**Tr.**	53
Cream Cheese	1 oz.	**1**	111
Cucumbers, raw	1–1¼″	**1**	5
Currants, raw	½ cup	**6**	25
Custard, baked	½ cup	**10**	114
boiled	½ cup	**13**	119
Custard Pie	1 medium slice	**34**	266
Dandelion Greens, raw	1 cup	**9**	44
cooked	½ cup	**6**	33
Dates	½ cup	**69**	274
Dehydrated Potato Flakes, milk and butter	3½ oz.	**15**	93
Doughnuts, plain	2	**40**	391
Dried Beef	3½ oz.	**0**	203
Duck	3½ oz.	**0**	165
Eel	3½ oz.	**0**	233
Eggplant	3½ oz.	**4**	19
Eggs, whole	1 medium	**Tr.**	72
white	1 medium	**Tr.**	15
yolk	1 medium	**Tr.**	57
Endive	3½ oz.	**4**	20
Evaporated Milk, canned	½ cup	**12**	138
Fats, vegetable fat, oil	1 tbs.	**0**	110
Fig Bars	1	**19**	85·5
Figs, raw	3 small	**20**	79

Food	Amount	Carbo-hydrate (grams)	Cals.
Figs, canned, syrup	½ cup	**22**	84
dried	3 small	**41**	165
Flounder, baked	3½ oz.	**0**	202
Frankfurter	1 medium	**1**	152
French Bread	3½ oz.	**55**	290
French Fried Potato	10 slices	**18**	137
French Salad Dressing	1 tbs.	**3**	63
Fruit Cake, dark	1 slice (2″×2″×½″)	**18**	118
Fruit Cocktail, canned	½ cup	**24**	60
Fudge, plain	3½ oz.	**81**	411
Gelatin, unflavoured	1 tbs.	**0**	34
Gelatin Dessert	½ cup	**14**	59
Gingerbread	2″ cube	**26**	163
Glacé Peel (lemon, orange, grapefruit)	3½ oz.	**81**	316
Gooseberries, raw	½ cup	**10·4**	40
Granulated Sugar, white	1 tbs.	**12**	48
Grapefruit, raw	½ small	**10**	40
canned	½ cup	**18**	70
Grapefruit Juice, fresh or frozen	½ cup	**9**	40
Grape Juice	½ cup	**21**	85
Grapes	3″ × 4″ bunch	**15**	70
Guavas	1 medium	**15**	62
Haddock, fried	3½ oz.	**7**	165
Halibut, broiled	3½ oz.	**0**	171
Ham	3½ oz.	**1**	340
Hamburger, broiled	3½ oz.	**0**	288
Hard Sweets	3½ oz.	**99**	383
Honey	1 tbs.	**17**	62
Honeydew Melon	1 medium slice	**8**	33
Ice Cream	¾ cup	**21**	207
Ice Milk	½ cup	**21**	116
Jams, preserves	1 tbs.	**14**	50
Jellies	1 tbs.	**13**	50
Kale, cooked	½ cup	**3·5**	20
Kidney Beans, canned or cooked	½ cup	**16**	90
Kidneys, beef	3½ oz.	**1**	130

Food	Amount	Carbo-hydrate (grams)	Cals.
Kidneys, pork	3½ oz.	**1**	106
Kohlrabi, cooked	⅔ cup	**7**	30
Lamb			
chop, broiled	3½ oz.	**0**	360
leg, roasted	3½ oz.	**0**	265
shoulder, roasted	3½ oz.	**0**	335
Lard	1 tbs.	**0**	126
Layer Cake, plain icing	3″ section	**60**	342
fudge icing	3″ section	**59**	349
Lemon Juice	½ cup	**8**	24
Lemons	1 medium	**8**	27
Lemon Meringue Pie	1 medium slice	**45**	302
Lemon Sole, steamed	3½ oz.	**0**	91
Lentils, mature	3½ oz.	**18**	106
Lettuce	¼ small head	**3**	13
	4 large leaves	**2**	18
Lima Beans, canned, drained	½ cup	**18**	96
cooked, fresh, or frozen	½ cup	**15**	85
Limburger Cheese	1 oz.	**1**	97
Lime Juice, fresh	¼ cup	**4·5**	12
Limes	1 medium	**5**	14
Liverwurst	3½ oz.	**2**	263
Lobster	3½ oz.	**Tr.**	95
Loganberries, raw	⅔ cup	**15**	62
Macaroni, cooked	⅔ cup	**30**	149
Malted Milk	1 cup	**32**	281
Margarine	1 tbs.	**Tr.**	101
Marshmallows	3½ oz.	**81**	325
Mayonnaise Salad Dressing	1 tbs.	**Tr.**	93
Milk, cows'			
whole	½ cup	**5·5**	68
skim	½ cup	**6**	36
canned, evaporated	½ cup	**12**	138
condensed	½ cup	**84**	490
dried, whole	1 tbs.	**3**	40
non-fat	1 tbs.	**4**	28
Milk, goats'	½ cup	**5**	67

Food	Amount	Carbo-hydrate (grams)	Cals.
Mince Pie	1 medium slice	62	341
Muffins	1 large	21	140
Mullet, steamed	3½ oz.	0	126
Mushrooms, raw	½ cup	4	28
canned, not drained	½ cup	2	17
Mushroom Soup, creamed	1 cup	17·5	220
Nectarines, raw	1 small	17	64
Noodles, egg, cooked	⅔ cup	23	125
Oatmeal, cooked	½ cup	13	75
Oils, cooking or salad	1 tbs.	0	124
Olives, green	10 large	2	70
ripe	10 large	2	125
Onions, raw	1 medium	9	38
cooked	½ cup	6	29
Onion Soup	1 cup	5	67
Orange Juice, fresh	½ cup	13	45
canned, unsweetened	½ cup	13	48
Oranges, peeled	1 small	15	49
Oysters, raw	5 medium	3	66
Oyster Stew, made with milk	1 cup	10	182
Pancakes, American, wheat, enriched	4 medium	27	218
buckwheat	4 medium	21	176
Parmesan Cheese	1 oz.	1	112
Parsley, raw	1 tbs.	Tr.	1
Parsnips, cooked	⅔ cup	15	66
Peaches, raw	1 small	10	38
canned, water	½ cup	8	31
canned, syrup	½ cup	20	78
frozen	3½ oz.	23	88
dried	⅔ cup	69	265
Peanut Brittle	3½ oz.	73	441
Peanut Butter	1 tbs.	3	43
Peanuts, roasted	⅔ cup	19	585
Pears, raw	1 medium	25	63
canned, water	½ cup	8	31
canned, syrup	1 medium	18	68
Peas, green, cooked, fresh, or frozen	⅔ cup	12	70
canned, drained	⅔ cup	17	58

Food	Amount	Carbo-hydrate (grams)	Cals.
Pea Soup	1 cup	25	130
Pecan nuts	½ cup	7·5	343
Peppers, green	1 large	5	25
Pickles			
Cucumber, dill	½ large	1	5·5
Cucumber, fresh (bread-and-butter type)	½ cup	17	70
Sour mixed	½ cup	2	11
Sweet mixed	½ cup	26	108
Pineapple, raw	¾ cup diced	14	52
canned, syrup	1 round slice	26	74
Pineapple Juice, unsweetened	½ cup	13	55
Pine Nuts (pignolia)	3½ oz.	12	552
Pistachio Nuts	3½ oz.	19	594
Plain cake, uniced	1 cupcake	29	164
iced	1 cupcake	31	161
Plums, raw	2 medium	13	50
canned, syrup	3 medium	25	112
Popcorn, popped	1 cup	10	54
Pork, fresh			
chops	1 small	0	260
roast, oven	3½ oz.	0	365
Pork Link Sausages	3½ oz.	0	476
Pork Liver, fried	3½ oz.	3	241
Pork Sausages, canned	3½ oz.	0	381
Potato Crisps	10 medium	10	114
Potato Flour	1 cup	80	351
Potatoes, baked	1 medium	21	93
boiled, peeled	1 medium	15	65
French fried	10 slices	18	137
mashed, milk and butter	½ cup	12	94
dehydrated flakes, milk and butter	3½ oz.	15	93
Pretzel Sticks	5 small	4	18
Prune Juice, canned	½ cup	21	77
Prunes, dried, raw	⅔ cup	67	255
cooked, unsweetened	⅔ cup	31	119
Prune Whip	¾ cup	37	148
Pumpkin Pie	1 medium slice	34	263

Food	Amount	Carbo-hydrate (grams)	Cals.
Radishes	2 small	0·5	3·5
Raisins	1 tbs.	7	29
Raspberries, red, raw	¾ cup	14	57
frozen, sweetened	½ cup	25	98
Rhubarb, raw	¾ cup	4	16
cooked, sweetened	⅔ cup	72	282
Rib of Beef, oven-roasted	3½ oz.	0	460
Rice, cooked, white	⅔ cup	24	109
Rice Cereals			
Flakes	1 cup	26	118
Krispies	1 cup	25	107
Puffed	1 cup	12	55
Rolls, plain	1 small	15	84
hamburger bun	1	21	118
Round Steak, broiled	3½ oz.	0	260
Round of Beef, oven-roasted	3½ oz.	0	260
Rye Flour	1¼ cups	75	350
Rye Bread	1 slice	12	57
Rye Wafers	1	5	21·5
Salmon, broiled	3½ oz.	0	182
canned	3½ oz.	0	210
smoked	3½ oz.	0	176
Sardines, canned, drained	3½ oz.	0	203
brine	3½ oz.	0	196
tomato sauce	3½ oz.	2	197
Sauerkraut, drained	⅔ cup	4	22
Scallops	3½ oz.	31	134
Shad, baked	3½ oz.	0	200
Sherbet	½ cup	31	134
Shredded Wheat	1 biscuit	23	102
Shrimp, fresh			
French fried	3½ oz.	10	225
canned, drained	3½ oz.	1	116
Sirloin, broiled	3½ oz.	0	390
Smelts, fried	3½ oz.	5	406
Snap Green Beans, cooked, fresh, frozen, canned, drained	¾ cup	5	25
Sole, fried	3½ oz.	5	273
Soybean Flour	½ cup	16·5	140
Soy Sauce	1 tbs.	1	10

Food	Amount	Carbo-hydrate (grams)	Cals.
Spaghetti, cooked	⅔ cup	**19**	149
Spinach, raw	3½ oz.	**4**	26
cooked	½ cup	**3**	23
Sponge Cake	1 large piece	**27**	195
Strawberries, raw	⅔ cup	**8**	37
frozen, sweetened	½ cup	**27**	106
Sugar			
Granulated, white	1 tbs.	**12**	48
Brown	1 tbs.	**13**	48
Sweet Potatoes, baked	1 small	**38**	141
boiled	½ medium	**26**	114
canned	½ cup	**25**	107
Swiss Cheese	1 oz.	**1**	105
Swiss Cheese, processed	1 oz.	**1**	101
Syrup	⅓ cup	**65**	252
Tangerine Juice, unsweetened, fresh, frozen, canned	½ cup	**11**	43
Tangerines	1 medium	**10**	46
Tapioca, dry	½ cup	**62·5**	264
Thousand Island Salad Dressing	1 tbs.	**2**	75
Tomatoes, raw	1 small	**5**	22
canned, cooked	½ cup	**4**	23
Tomato Juice	½ cup	**5**	19
Tomato Ketchup	1 tbs.	**4**	17
Tomato Soup, creamed	1 cup	**5**	67
Tongue, beef	3½ oz.	**Tr.**	240
Treacle	⅓ cup	**60**	232
Trout, steamed	3½ oz.	**0**	133
Tuna Fish, canned, drained	3½ oz.	**0**	198
Turbot, steamed	3½ oz.	**0**	98
Turkey	3½ oz.	**0**	190
Turnip Greens	⅔ cup	**4**	20
Turnips, raw, diced	¾ cup	**7**	30
Veal, cutlet	3½ oz.	**0**	220
roast	3½ oz.	**0**	360
braised	3½ oz.	**0**	303
Vegetable with Beef Soup	1 cup	**10**	80
Vienna Bread	3½ oz.	**55**	290
Vienna Sausages, canned	3½ oz.	**3**	81

Food	Amount	Carbo-hydrate (grams)	Cals.
Vinegar	¼ cup	2·5	6
Waffles	1 large	31	275
Walnuts	1 tbs. chopped	1	52
	½ cup halves	8	325
Watermelon	¾″ × 8–10″ slice	11	45
Wheat Flours			
white	½ cup	38	132
whole wheat	½ cup	35·5	166·5
Wheat Germ	3½ oz.	47	363
White Bread	1 small slice	12	37
White Sauce	½ cup	9	162
Whole Wheat Bread	1 small slice	11	60
Yeast, brewers'	1 tbs.	3	22
Yoghurt	½ cup	12·5	60

TABLE OF FOOD VALUES IN COMMON PORTIONS

[by categories]

Amounts of food on this table refer to edible portions only. All spoonful measurements are level. All cup and portion of cup measurements are scant unless otherwise cited. Fruit measurements include skin unless otherwise noted. Please note that caloric values, which have no significance in the low carbohydrate diet, have been included here purely as a point of interest and comparison for the curious.

Food	Amount	Carbohydrate (grams)	Cals.
BREADS			
Bread Crumbs	1 cup	**72**	385
Breads			
Brown	1 small slice	**23**	105
French or Vienna	3½ oz.	**55**	290
Rye	1 small slice	**12**	57
White	1 small slice	**12**	57
Whole wheat, entire wheat	1 small slice	**11**	60
Crackers			
Saltine	2 whole	**6**	34
Soda	1 medium	**4**	22
Muffins	1 large	**21**	140
Pancakes, American			
wheat, enriched	4 medium	**27**	218
buckwheat	4 medium	**21**	176
Pretzel Sticks	5 small	**4**	18
Rolls, plain	1 small	**15**	84
hamburger bun	1	**21**	118

Food	Amount	Carbo-hydrate (grams)	Cals.
Rye Wafers	1	**5**	21·5
Waffles	1 large	**31**	275
CEREALS			
Barley	½ cup	**79**	349
Corn Flakes	1 cup	**21**	95
Cornmeal, all kinds	½ cup	**11**	50
Cornstarch	1 tbs.	**7**	29
Macaroni, cooked	⅔ cup	**30**	149
Noodles, egg, cooked	⅔ cup	**23**	125
Oatmeal, cooked	½ cup	**13**	75
Popcorn, popped	1 cup	**10**	54
Potato Flour	1 cup	**80**	351
Rice, cooked, white	⅔ cup	**24**	109
Rice cereals			
Flakes	1 cup	**26**	118
Krispies	1 cup	**25**	107
Puffed	1 cup	**12**	55
Rye Flour	1¼ cups	**75**	350
Shredded Wheat	1 biscuit	**23**	102
Soybean Flour	½ cup	**16·5**	140
Spaghetti, cooked	⅔ cup	**19**	149
Wheat Flours			
white	½ cup	**38**	132
whole wheat	½ cup	**35·5**	166·5
Wheat Germ	3½ oz.	**47**	363
Yeast, brewers'	1 tbs.	**3**	22
DRESSINGS AND CONDIMENTS, FATS			
Butter	1 tbs.	**Tr.**	100
Chilli Sauce	1 tbs.	**4**	17
Fats, vegetable fat, oil	1 tbs.	**0**	110
Lard	1 tbs.	**0**	126
Margarine	1 tbs.	**Tr.**	101
Oils, cooking or salad	1 tbs.	**0**	124
Peanut Butter	1 tbs.	**3**	43
Salad Dressings, French	1 tbs.	**3**	63
Mayonnaise	1 tbs.	**Tr.**	93
Thousand Island	1 tbs.	**2**	75

Food	Amount	Carbo-hydrate (grams)	Cals.
Soy Sauce	1 tbs.	1	10
Tomato Ketchup	1 tbs.	4	17
Vinegar	¼ cup	2·5	6
White Sauce	½ cup	9	162
FISH AND SHELLFISH			
Fish			
Cod, broiled	3½ oz.	0	170
dried	3½ oz.	0	375
Eel	3½ oz.	0	233
Flounder, baked	3½ oz.	0	202
Haddock, fried	3½ oz.	7	165
Halibut, broiled	3½ oz.	0	171
Lemon Sole, steamed	3½ oz.	0	91
Mullet, steamed	3½ oz.	0	126
Salmon, broiled	3½ oz.	0	182
canned	3½ oz.	0	210
smoked	3½ oz.	0	176
Sardines, canned, drained	3½ oz.	0	203
tomato sauce	3½ oz.	2	197
Shad, baked	3½ oz.	0	200
Smelts, fried	3½ oz.	5	406
Sole, fried	3½ oz.	5	273
Trout, steamed	3½ oz.	0	133
Tuna Fish, canned, drained	3½ oz.	0	198
Turbot, steamed	3½ oz.	0	98
Shellfish			
Clams, canned, undrained	3½ oz.	3	51
Crab, hard shell, canned or cooked	3½ oz.	1	101
Lobster	3½ oz.	Tr.	95
Oysters, raw	5 medium	3	66
Scallops	3½ oz.	3	81
Shrimp, fresh	3 oz.	0	110
French fried	3½ oz.	10	225
canned, drained	3½ oz.	1	116
FRUIT			
Apple, raw	1 small	15	58
frozen, sliced, sweetened	⅔ cup	24	92

Food	Amount	Carbo-hydrate (grams)	Cals.
Apple sauce, unsweetened	½ cup	12	42
Apricots, raw	3 medium	13	51
canned, water	½ cup	10	38
canned, syrup	½ cup	22	86
dried, uncooked	5 medium halves	13	52
cooked, unsweetened	½ cup	31	183
frozen	½ cup	25	98
Avocados	half, peeled	6	167
Bananas	1 small	22	85
Berries			
Blackberries			
raw	½ cup	9	40
canned, water	½ cup	9	43
canned, syrup	½ cup	22	91
Blueberries,			
raw	⅔ cup	15	61
frozen, no sugar	⅔ cup	14	56
canned, water	½ cup	10	37
canned, syrup	½ cup	26	98
Cranberries, raw	½ cup	6	23
canned, strained	½ cup	38	146
Gooseberries, raw	½ cup	10·4	40
Loganberries, raw	⅔ cup	15	62
Raspberries, red, raw	¾ cup	14	57
frozen, sweetened	½ cup	25	98
Strawberries, raw	⅔ cup	8	37
frozen, sweetened	½ cup	27	106
Cantaloupe	½ melon	8	30
Cherries, raw	½ cup	8	32
canned, sour red	½ cup	15	60
Currants, raw	½ cup	6	25
Dates	½ cup	69	274
Figs, raw	3 small	20	79
canned, syrup	½ cup	22	84
dried	3 small	41	165
Grapefruit, fresh	½ small	10	40
canned	½ cup	18	70
Grapes	3″ × 4″ bunch	15	70

Food	Amount	Carbo-hydrate (grams)	Cals.
Guavas	1 medium	15	62
Honeydew Melon	1 medium slice	8	33
Lemons	1 medium	8	27
Limes	1 medium	5	14
Nectarines, raw	1 small	17	64
Oranges, peeled	1 small	15	49
Peaches, raw	1 small	10	38
canned, water	½ cup	8	31
canned, syrup	½ cup	20	78
frozen	3½ oz.	23	88
dried	⅔ cup	69	265
Pears, raw	1 medium	25	63
canned, water	½ cup	8	31
canned, syrup	1 medium	18	68
Pineapple, raw	¾ cup diced	14	52
canned, syrup	1 round slice	26	74
Plums, raw	2 medium	13	50
canned, syrup	3 medium	25	112
Prunes, dried, raw	⅔ cup	67	255
cooked, unsweetened	⅔ cup	31	119
cooked, sweetened	⅔ cup	45	172
Raisins	1 tbs.	7	29
Rhubarb, raw	¾ cup	4	16
cooked, sweetened	⅔ cup	72	282
Tangerines	1 medium	10	46
Watermelon	¾″ × 8–10″ slice	11	45
JUICES			
Apple juice	½ cup	17	47
Grapefruit juice, fresh or frozen	½ cup	9	40
Grape juice	½ cup	21	85
Lemon juice	½ cup	8	24
Lime juice, fresh	¼ cup	4·5	12
Orange juice, fresh	½ cup	13	45
canned, unsweetened	½ cup	13	48
frozen, reconstituted	½ cup	13	45

Food	Amount	Carbo-hydrate (grams)	Cals.
Pineapple juice, unsweetened	½ cup	13	55
Prune juice, canned	½ cup	21	77
Tangerine juice, unsweetened,	½ cup	11	43
Tomato juice	½ cup	5	19
MEAT			
Bacon	2 strips	Tr.	97
Beef, various cuts braised, pot-roasted, lean and fat	3½ oz.	0	288
hamburger, broiled	3½ oz.	0	288
oven roasted, rib	3½ oz.	0	460
steak, broiled, sirloin	3½ oz.	0	390
round (relatively lean)	3½ oz.	0	260
canned, corned beef	3½ oz.	0	212
corned beef hash	3½ oz.	7	140
chopped, creamed	3½ oz.	7	154
dried	3½ oz.	0	203
stew (with veg.)	½ cup	7	107
Brains, calves', boiled	3½ oz.	1	102
Kidneys, beef	3½ oz.	1	130
pork	3½ oz.	1	106
Lamb			
chop, broiled	3½ oz.	0	360
leg, roasted	3½ oz.	0	265
shoulder, roasted	3½ oz.	0	335
Liver			
beef, fried	3½ oz.	5	229
calf, fried	3½ oz.	4	261
chicken, cooked	3½ oz.	3	165
pork, fried	3½ oz.	3	241
Pork, fresh			
chops	1 small chop	0	260
roast, oven	3½ oz.	0	365
simmered	3½ oz.	0	375
smoked, cured ham	3½ oz.	1	340
Sausages, bologna	3½ oz.	7	300
frankfurter	1 medium	1	152
liverwurst	3½ oz.	2	263
pork links	3½ oz.	0	476

Food	Amount	Carbo-hydrate (grams)	Cals.
Sausages, pork, canned	3½ oz.	0	381
Vienna, canned	3½ oz.	0	240
Tongue, beef	3½ oz.	Tr.	240
Veal, cutlet	3½ oz.	0	220
roast	3½ oz.	0	360
braised	3½ oz.	0	303
MILK AND MILK PRODUCTS			
Buttermilk	½ cup	5	36
Cheese			
Blue	1 oz.	1	104
Camembert	1 oz.	1	85
Cheddar	1 oz.	1	113
Cheddar, processed	1 oz.	1	105
Cottage, uncreamed	1 oz.	1	26
Cream	1 oz.	1	111
Limburger	1 oz.	1	97
Parmesan	1 oz.	1	112
Swiss	1 oz.	1	105
Swiss, processed	1 oz.	1	101
Cream			
light	1 tbs.	1	31
heavy	1 tbs.	Tr.	53
sour	1 tbs.	Tr.	53
Ice Cream	¾ cup	21	207
Milk Beverages			
Malted	1 cup	32	281
Chocolate	1 cup	22	148
Cocoa	1 cup	27	236
Milk, cows'			
whole	½ cup	5·5	68
skim	½ cup	6	36
Milk, canned			
evaporated	½ cup	12	138
condensed	½ cup	84	490
Milk, dried			
whole	1 tbs.	3	40
non-fat	1 tbs.	4	28
Milk, goats'	½ cup	5	67
Yoghurt	½ cup	12·5	60

Food	Amount	Carbohydrate (grams)	Cals.
NUTS			
Almonds	12–15	5	90
Brazil Nuts	⅔ cup	11	654
Cashew Nuts	¼ cup	9	168
Coconut			
fresh, shredded	½ cup	4·5	173
dried, shredded, sweetened	½ cup	16·5	173
Peanuts, roasted	⅔ cup	19	585
Pecans	½ cup	7·5	343
Pine Nuts (pignolia)	3½ oz.	12	552
Pistachio Nuts	3½ oz.	19	594
Walnuts, chopped	1 tbs.	1	52
halves	½ cup	8	325
POULTRY AND PRODUCTS			
Chicken, broiled	3½ oz.	0	218
Duck	3½ oz.	0	165
Turkey	3½ oz.	0	190
Eggs			
whole	1 medium	Tr.	72
white	1 medium	Tr.	15
yolk	1 medium	Tr.	57
SOUPS			
Bouillon Cubes	1	Tr.	2
Soups, canned			
Beef Bouillon	1 cup	0	32
Chicken Noodle	1 cup	7·5	65
Clam Chowder	1 cup	12·5	82
Onion	1 cup	5	67
Oyster Stew made with milk	1 cup	10	182
Pea	1 cup	25	130
Vegetable with Beef	1 cup	10	80
Creamed			
Celery	1 cup	17·5	162
Chicken	1 cup	15	182
Mushroom	1 cup	17·5	220
Tomato	1 cup	15	90

Food	Amount	Carbo-hydrate (grams)	Cals.
SWEETS AND DESSERTS			
Cake			
Angel Food	2″ section	**24**	**108**
Cupcake, uniced	1 cupcake	**29**	**164**
iced	1 cupcake	**31**	**161**
Fruit, dark	1 slice (2″×2″×½″)	**18**	**118**
Layer cake, plain icing	3″ section	**60**	**342**
fudge icing	3″ section	**59**	**349**
Sponge	1 large piece	**27**	**195**
Chocolate, bitter	1 oz.	**8**	**142**
bittersweet	1 oz.	**14**	**143**
Chocolate sauce	1 tbs.	**13**	**49**
Custard, baked	½ cup	**10**	**114**
boiled	½ cup	**13**	**119**
Doughnuts, plain	2	**40**	**391**
Fig Bars	1	**19**	85·5
Fruit Cocktail, canned	½ cup	**24**	**60**
Gelatin, unflavoured	1 tbs.	**0**	**34**
Gelatin dessert	½ cup	**14**	**59**
Gingerbread	2″ cube	**26**	**163**
Honey	1 tbs.	**17**	**62**
Jams, preserves	1 tbs.	**14**	**50**
Jellies	1 tbs.	**13**	**50**
Pies			
Apple	1 medium slice	**53**	**331**
Blueberry	1 medium slice	**51**	**291**
Cherry	1 medium slice	**55**	**340**
Custard	1 medium slice	**34**	**266**
Lemon meringue	1 medium slice	**45**	**302**
Mince	1 medium slice	**62**	**341**
Pumpkin	1 medium slice	**34**	**263**

Food	Amount	Carbo-hydrate (grams)	Cals.
Prune Whip	¾ cup	**37**	148
Sherbet	½ cup	**31**	134
Sugar, granulated, white	1 tbs.	**12**	48
brown	1 tbs.	**13**	48
Sweets			
Butterscotch	3½ oz.	**86**	410
Caramels	3½ oz.	**78**	415
Chocolate, milk	1 oz.	**16**	143
Chocolate, milk with almonds	1 oz.	**14**	151
Fudge, plain	3⅓ oz.	**81**	411
Glacé-peel (lemon, orange, grape-fruit)	3½ oz.	**81**	316
Hard sweets	3½ oz.	**99**	383
Marshmallows	3½ oz.	**81**	325
Peanut Brittle	3½ oz.	**73**	441
Syrup	⅓ cup	**65**	252
Treacle	⅓ cup	**60**	232
VEGETABLES			
Artichokes, Globe, boiled	1 medium	**5·5**	8
Jerusalem, boiled	1 oz.	**0·9**	5
Asparagus, cooked, fresh or frozen	6–7 spears	**4**	20
canned, drained	6–7 spears	**3**	21
Beans			
Common, kidney, canned or cooked	½ cup	**16**	90
Lima, cooked, fresh or frozen	½ cup	**15**	85
canned, drained	½ cup	**18**	96
Snap green, cooked, fresh or frozen	¾ cup	**5**	24
Bean sprouts	½ cup	**3·5**	17·5
Beetroot, cooked or canned, drained	½ cup	**9**	35
Broccoli, cooked	⅔ cup	**5**	26
Brussels sprouts	¾ cup	**7**	36
Cabbage, raw	3″ × 4″ portion	**5**	24
cooked	1⅔ cup	**4**	20
Carrots, raw	1 medium	**4·5**	21
cooked, drained	½ cup	**5**	22
canned, drained	½ cup	**5**	22

Food	Amount	Carbo-hydrate (grams)	Cals.
Cauliflower, raw	½ cup	**3**	15·5
cooked, drained	½ cup	**3**	15
Celery, raw	½ cup diced	**2**	12
cooked, drained	½ cup diced	**2·5**	17
Corn, fresh, cooked	1 small ear	**18**	91
canned, cream style	½ cup	**20**	82
canned, whole kernel	½ cup	**16**	66
Cucumbers, raw	1–1¼″	**1**	5
Dandelion Greens, raw	1 cup	**9**	44
cooked	½ cup	**6**	33
Eggplant	3½ oz.	**4**	19
Endive	3½ oz.	**4**	20
Kale, cooked	½ cup	**3·5**	20
Kohlrabi, cooked	⅔ cup	**7**	30
Lentils, mature	3½ oz.	**18**	106
Lettuce	¼ small head	**3**	13
	4 large leaves	**2**	18
Mushrooms, raw	½ cup	**4**	28
canned, not drained	½ cup	**2**	17
Olives, green	10 large	**2**	70
Onions, raw	1 medium	**9**	38
cooked	½ cup	**6**	29
Parsley, raw	1 tbs.	**Tr.**	1
Parsnips, cooked	⅔ cup	**15**	66
Peas, green cooked, fresh or frozen	⅔ cup	**12**	70
canned, drained	⅔ cup	**17**	58
Peppers, green	1 large	**5**	25
Pickles			
Cucumber, dill	½ large	**1**	5·5
Cucumber, fresh (bread-and-butter type)	½ cup	**17**	70
Sour mixed	½ cup	**2**	11
Sweet mixed	½ cup	**26**	108
Potatoes, baked	1 medium	**21**	93
boiled, peeled	1 medium	**15**	65
French fried	10 slices	**18**	137
mashed (milk and butter)	½ cup	**12**	94
dehydrated flakes (milk and butter)	3½ oz.	**15**	93

Food	Amount	Carbo-hydrate (grams)	Cals.
Potato Crisps	10 medium	**10**	114
Radishes	2 small	**0·5**	3·5
Sauerkraut, drained	⅔ cup	**4**	22
Spinach, raw	3½ oz.	**4**	26
cooked	½ cup	**3**	23
Sweet Potatoes, baked	1 small	**38**	141
boiled	½ medium	**26**	114
canned	½ cup	**25**	107
Tomatoes, raw	1 small	**5**	22
canned, cooked	½ cup	**4**	23
Turnip Greens	⅔ cup	**4**	20
Turnips, raw, diced	¾ cup	**7**	30
boiled, drained	⅔ cup	**5**	23

CARBOHYDRATE CONTENT OF COMMON SNACKS

Snack	Amount	Carbohydrate (grams)
Almonds	10	**2**
Anchovy paste	1 tbs.	**Trace**
Blue cheese spread	1 oz.	**1**
Bluemould (Roquefort) cheese	1 1″ cube	**Trace**
Camembert cheese	1 1″ cube	**Trace**
Cashew nuts	6	**3**
Caviar on toast	2″ square	**3**
Cheddar cheese	1 1″ cube	**Trace**
Cocktail sausages	each	**Trace**
Cottage cheese	2 tbs.	**1**
Cream cheese	1 1″ cube	**Trace**
Green olives	10 large	**2**
Gruyère cheese	1 1″ cube	**Trace**
Liederkranz cheese	1 1″ cube	**Trace**
Limburger cheese	1 1″ cube	**Trace**
Parmesan cheese	1 1″ cube	**1**
Pâté de foie gras	1 tbs.	**Trace**
Peanuts, roasted, salted	30	**4**
Pickled, raw herring	1 serving	**0**
Pimento cheese spread	1 oz.	**1**
Potato crisps	5 medium	**5**
Raw carrot sticks	3 thin	**3**
Ripe olives	10 large	**2**
Roast turkey slices	1 serving	**0**
Shrimp, plain	1 serving	**Trace**
Smoked ham	1 serving	**Trace**
Swiss cheese	1 1″ cube	**Trace**

CARBOHYDRATE CONTENT OF BEVERAGES

Beverage	Amount	Carbohydrate (grams)
Apple juice	½ cup	**17**
Apricot nectar	½ cup	**18**
Cider, sweet	1 cup	**34**
Coffee or tea		**0**
Cola drinks (with sugar)	1 cup	**28**
Cranberry juice	½ cup	**18**
Ginger Ale	1 cup	**21**
Grapefruit juice	½ cup	**12**
Grape juice	½ cup	**21**
Lemonade, frozen	½ cup	**14**
Low calorie soft drinks		**0**
Orange juice, unsweetened	½ cup	**13**
Peach nectar	½ cup	**15·5**
Pear nectar	½ cup	**16·5**
Pineapple juice, unsweetened	½ cup	**13**
Prune juice	½ cup	**21**
Soda water		**0**
Tangerine juice, unsweetened	½ cup	**11**
Tomato juice	½ cup	**5**
Water		**0**

CARBOHYDRATE CONTENT OF ALCOHOLIC BEVERAGES

Alcoholic Beverage	Amount	Carbohydrate (grams)
Ale, mild	12 oz.	12
Anisette	1 oz.	7
Apricot Brandy	1 oz.	6
Beer, lager	12 oz.	18
Benedictine	1 oz.	7
Champagne, dry	4 oz.	2
Cider, hard	6 oz.	2
Crème de Menthe	1 oz.	6
Curacao	1 oz.	6
Daiquiri	3 oz.	5
Distilled spirits (whisky, gin, vodka, rum, brandy)	1 oz.	Trace
Eggnog	4 oz.	18
Gin and Tonic	10 oz.	9
Manhattan	3 oz.	7
Martini	3 oz.	Trace
Mint Julep	10 oz.	3
Muscatel	2 oz.	7
Old Fashioned	4 oz.	4
Planter's Punch	10 oz.	8
Port	2 oz.	7
Sherry, dry	2 oz.	1
Sherry, medium	2 oz.	2
Sherry, sweet	2 oz.	6
Tom Collins	10 oz.	9
Vermouth, French	3 oz.	4
Vermouth, Italian	3 oz.	14
Vodka		0
Wine, dry white	4 oz.	Trace
Wine, red	4 oz.	Trace
Wine, rosé	4 oz	1

DESIRABLE WEIGHTS FOR ADULTS

MEN	FRAME		
	Small	Medium	Large
5 feet 2 inches	8 st. 3 lb. – 8 st. 11 lb.	8 st. 9 lb. – 9 st. 7 lb.	9 st. 3 lb. –10 st. 4 lb.
5 feet 3 inches	8 st. 6 lb. – 9 st.	8 st. 12 lb.– 9 st. 10 lb.	9 st. 6 lb. –10 st. 8 lb.
5 feet 4 inches	8 st. 9 lb. – 9 st. 3 lb.	9 st. 1 lb. – 9 st. 13 lb.	9 st. 9 lb. –10 st. 12 lb.
5 feet 5 inches	8 st. 12 lb.– 9 st. 7 lb.	9 st. 4 lb. –10 st. 3 lb.	9 st. 12 lb.–11 st. 2 lb.
5 feet 6 inches	9 st. 2 lb. – 9 st. 11 lb.	9 st. 8 lb. –10 st. 7 lb.	10 st. 2 lb. –11 st. 7 lb.
5 feet 7 inches	9 st. 6 lb. –10 st. 1 lb.	9 st. 12 lb.–10 st. 12 lb.	10 st. 7 lb. –11 st. 12 lb.
5 feet 8 inches	9 st. 10 lb.–10 st. 5 lb.	10 st. 2 lb. –11 st. 2 lb.	10 st. 11 lb.–12 st. 2 lb.
5 feet 9 inches	10 st. –10 st. 10 lb.	10 st. 6 lb. –11 st. 6 lb.	11 st. 1 lb. –12 st. 6 lb.
5 feet 10 inches	10 st. 4 lb. –11 st.	10 st. 10 lb.–11 st. 11 lb.	11 st. 5 lb. –12 st. 11 lb.
5 feet 11 inches	10 st. 8 lb. –11 st. 4 lb.	11 st. –12 st. 2 lb.	11 st. 10 lb.–13 st. 2 lb.
6 feet 0 inches	10 st. 12 lb.–11 st. 8 lb.	11 st. 4 lb. –12 st. 7 lb.	12 st. –13 st. 7 lb.
6 feet 1 inch	11 st. 2 lb. –11 st. 13 lb.	11 st. 8 lb. –12 st. 12 lb.	12 st. 5 lb. –13 st. 12 lb.
6 feet 2 inches	11 st. 6 lb. –12 st. 3 lb.	11 st. 13 lb.–13 st. 3 lb.	12 st. 10 lb.–14 st. 3 lb.

WOMEN	FRAME		
	Small	Medium	Large
4 feet 10 inches	6 st. 12 lb.– 7 st. 6 lb.	7 st. 3 lb. – 8 st. 1 lb.	7 st. 11 lb.– 8 st. 13 lb.
4 feet 11 inches	7 st. 1 lb. – 7 st. 9 lb.	7 st. 6 lb. – 8 st. 4 lb.	8 st. – 9 st. 2 lb.
5 feet 0 inches	7 st. 4 lb. – 7 st. 12 lb.	7 st. 9 lb. – 8 st. 7 lb.	8 st. 3 lb. – 9 st. 5 lb.
5 feet 1 inch	7 st. 7 lb. – 8 st. 1 lb.	7 st. 12 lb.– 8 st. 10 lb.	8 st. 6 lb. – 9 st. 8 lb.
5 feet 2 inches	7 st. 10 lb.– 8 st. 4 lb.	8 st. 1 lb. – 9 st.	8 st. 9 lb. – 9 st. 12 lb.
5 feet 3 inches	7 st. 13 lb.– 8 st. 7 lb.	8 st. 4 lb. – 9 st. 4 lb.	8 st. 13 lb.–10 st. 2 lb.
5 feet 4 inches	8 st. 2 lb. – 8 st. 11 lb.	8 st. 8 lb. – 9 st. 9 lb.	9 st. 3 lb. –10 st. 6 lb.
5 feet 5 inches	8 st. 6 lb. – 9 st. 1 lb.	8 st. 12 lb.– 9 st. 13 lb.	9 st. 7 lb. –10 st. 10 lb.
5 feet 6 inches	8 st. 10 lb.– 9 st. 5 lb.	9 st. 2 lb. –10 st. 3 lb.	9 st. 11 lb.–11 st.
5 feet 7 inches	9 st. – 9 st. 9 lb.	9 st. 6 lb. –10 st. 7 lb.	10 st. 1 lb. –11 st. 4 lb.
5 feet 8 inches	9 st. 4 lb. –10 st.	9 st. 10 lb.–10 st. 11 lb.	10 st. 5 lb. –11 st. 9 lb.
5 feet 9 inches	9 st. 8 lb. –10 st. 4 lb.	10 st. –11 st. 1 lb.	10 st. 9 lb. –12 st.
5 feet 10 inches	9 st. 12 lb.–10 st. 8 lb.	10 st. 4 lb. –11 st. 5 lb.	10 st. 13 lb.–12 st. 5 lb.

LOW CARBOHYDRATE DIET MENUS

Beverages at all meals: coffee or tea with as much cream as desired and artificial sweetener. Recipes for many of the dishes in these menus can be found in the section following.

BREAKFAST— 22 grams	LUNCH— 9 grams	DINNER— 25·5 grams
½ cup blueberries with cream Poached egg and ham on slice of buttered toast	Chicken salad in avocado half Lettuce wedge with mayonnaise	Lamb with radish sauce Salad of artichoke heart and endive 1 dessert pancake with jam
TOTAL FOR THE DAY: 56·5 grams		

BREAKFAST— 21 grams	LUNCH— 11 grams	DINNER— 25·5 grams
½ cup grapefruit juice Herb omelette Bacon 1 thin slice buttered toast	Poached halibut and mayonnaise Cucumber salad 2 soda crackers Cheese	Chicken with curry cream Lemon-buttered asparagus Small slice dark fruit cake (without dates)
TOTAL FOR THE DAY: 57·5 grams		

BREAKFAST— 24 grams	LUNCH— 18 grams	DINNER— 16 grams
½ cup water-packed canned pears, drained Liver and bacon 1 thin slice buttered toast	Broiled steak Asparagus vinaigrette Thin slice sponge cake	Parma veal Carrots steamed in butter Slice of honeydew melon
TOTAL FOR THE DAY: 58 grams		

BREAKFAST— 19 grams	LUNCH— 6 grams	DINNER— 29 grams
½ cup strawberries with cream 2 soft-boiled eggs 1 thin slice buttered toast	Broiled chopped beef patty Sliced tomatoes and cucumber salad	Chicken breasts à la Suisse Broccoli with butter Green salad with plain dressing Slice of cheese Small bunch of grapes

TOTAL FOR THE DAY: 54 grams

BREAKFAST— 19·5 grams	LUNCH— 14 grams	DINNER— 23 grams
½ navel orange, in sections Eggs scrambled with cream Bacon 1 thin slice buttered white toast	Cold roast beef Cabbage salad 2 soda crackers Slice of cheese	Baked flounder Ning Po spinach Half avocado, French dressing Lemon chiffon pudding

TOTAL FOR THE DAY: 56·5 grams

BREAKFAST— 28 grams	LUNCH— 15 grams	DINNER— 9·4 grams
½ grapefruit Sautéed kidney and mushrooms with ham 1 slice toast	Tomato juice Tuna fish salad 10 potato crisps	Pork chops Charcutière Sautéed cabbage Coffee fluff

TOTAL FOR THE DAY: 52·4 grams

BREAKFAST— 21 grams	LUNCH— 13 grams	DINNER— 15·5 grams
Slice of honeydew melon Eggs scrambled with salami 1 thin slice buttered toast	½ avocado stuffed with shrimp salad 2 slices tomato 1 thin slice Angel Food cake	Veal kidneys with mustard sauce Cauliflower Slice of cheese 2 soda crackers

TOTAL FOR THE DAY: 49·5 grams

BREAKFAST— 13 grams	LUNCH— 14 grams	DINNER— 31 grams
Baked eggs in cream 1 thin slice buttered toast	Sardines Green salad with dill and cucumber 10 medium potato crisps Slice of cheese	Mock boar ½ cup rice Strawberries with kirsch

TOTAL FOR THE DAY: 58 grams

BREAKFAST— 12 grams	LUNCH— 27 grams	DINNER— 13 grams
2 fried eggs Bacon 1 thin slice buttered toast	Chile rellenos and Mexican sauce 1 small fresh pear	Hamburgers with Bordelaise sauce ½ cup beetroot vinaigrette Coffee fluff

TOTAL FOR THE DAY: 52 grams

BREAKFAST— 17 grams	LUNCH— 27 grams	DINNER— 10 grams
½ cup tomato juice Steamed turbot slice of lemon 1 thin slice buttered rye toast	Chicken consommé with spinach and poached egg 2 soda crackers ½ cup ice cream	Leg of lamb, roasted— basted with red wine Broccoli Endive salad Slice of cheese

TOTAL FOR THE DAY: 54 grams

BREAKFAST— 29 grams	LUNCH— 14 grams	DINNER— 13 grams
½ cup grapefruit juice Ham slice sprinkled with 1 tsp. brown sugar and nutmeg and grilled 1 small roll	Baked shad Asparagus with Hollandaise sauce Apricot whip (with artificial sweetener)	Garlic chicken Cucumber salad Baked custard

TOTAL FOR THE DAY: 56 grams

BREAKFAST— 20 grams	LUNCH— 15·5 grams	DINNER— 23 grams
½ cup fresh strawberries with cream 2 soft-boiled eggs 2 slices bacon 1 thin slice buttered toast	Cold chicken 10 slices French-fried potatoes Cabbage salad	Pork roast ½ cup Brussels sprouts Small slice dark fruit cake

TOTAL FOR THE DAY: 58·5 grams

BREAKFAST— 25 grams	LUNCH— 10·5 grams	DINNER— 23·5 grams
½ cup grapefruit juice Fried liver and bacon 1 thin slice buttered toast	Baked Eggs with Anchovy ½ broiled tomato 1 soda cracker with cheese	Stuffed chicken breasts, Kiev style Green beans, Hollandaise ½ cup applesauce with artificial sweetener, topped with whipped cream and chopped nuts

TOTAL FOR THE DAY: 59 grams

BREAKFAST— 13 grams	LUNCH— 15 grams	DINNER— 31 grams
Cheese omelette 1 thin slice buttered toast	2 lamb chops Green salad ½ small canned pear, drained, with fresh coconut	Orient beef ½ cup boiled thin egg noodles Slice of cheese

TOTAL FOR THE DAY: 59 grams

BREAKFAST— 21 grams	LUNCH— 24·5 grams	DINNER— 14·5 grams
½ cup grapefruit juice 2 fried eggs with pork sausage 1 thin slice buttered rye toast	Chicken noodle soup 1 slice protein toast cut into fingers, spread with cream cheese Baked custard made with artificial sweetener	Lamb Shanks Brazil Stewed green pepper ½ cup water-packed canned blackberries

TOTAL FOR THE DAY: 60 grams

BREAKFAST— 17 grams	LUNCH— 22 grams	DINNER— 17 grams
½ cup tomato juice 2 eggs scrambled with sausages 1 thin slice buttered toast	Chicken salad in avocado half 1 small roll with cream cheese	Broiled or boiled lobster with drawn butter 10 pieces of French-fried potatoes Green salad Coffee fluff

TOTAL FOR THE DAY: 56 grams

BREAKFAST— 21 grams	LUNCH— 25 grams	DINNER— 10 grams
½ cup grapefruit juice 2 boiled eggs 1 thin slice buttered whole wheat toast	Grilled cheese and bacon sandwich on thin-sliced bread	Broiled steak Canned asparagus served with butter Slice of honeydew melon

TOTAL FOR THE DAY: 56 grams

BREAKFAST— 18 grams	LUNCH— 16 grams	DINNER— 25 grams
½ cup fresh strawberries 2 fried eggs 1 thin slice buttered toast	Chef's salad—cheese, ham, cold chicken with Roquefort dressing 1 slice Melba toast Slice of honeydew melon	Butter broiled chicken Green beans and tiny white onions with cream ½ cup unsweetened applesauce with Cointreau-flavoured whipped cream

TOTAL FOR THE DAY: 59 grams

BREAKFAST— 22 grams	LUNCH— 7 grams	DINNER— 30 grams
½ grapefruit 2 poached eggs on 1 thin slice buttered toast 2 strips bacon	Fried sausage with 2 fried apple rings 1 soda cracker with cream cheese	Roast duckling with giblet sauce Sautéed turnips ½ canned pear, light syrup pack, drained, with 1 tbs. chocolate sauce (semi-sweet chips melted in heavy cream)

TOTAL FOR THE DAY: 59 grams

BREAKFAST— 17 grams	LUNCH— 21 grams	DINNER— 16 grams
½ cup tomato juice Scrambled eggs and bacon 1 thin slice buttered toast	½ cantaloupe Cold beef Mustard pickles Slice of cheese 2 soda crackers	Broiled steak ½ cup spinach with butter or cream Small portion mashed potato Custard Crème

TOTAL FOR THE DAY: 54 grams

BREAKFAST— 13 grams	LUNCH— 15·5 grams	DINNER— 30·5 grams
Grilled ham with poached egg 1 thin slice buttered toast	Broiled chopped beef patty 2 slices herb-sprinkled tomato 10 slices French-fried potatoes	Fegato Agrodolce ⅓ cup boiled egg noodles Cucumber with sour cream and chives Slice of cheese 2 soda crackers

TOTAL FOR THE DAY: 59 grams

BREAKFAST— 22 grams	LUNCH— 10 grams	DINNER— 23 grams
½ grapefruit 2 small American pancakes with butter	Clear onion soup with grated cheese Lemon sole, fried Coffee gelatin made with artificial sweetener	Chicken with Fennel green beans with brown butter garlic sauce ½ cup ice cream sprinkled with ¼ cup fresh coconut

TOTAL FOR THE DAY: 55 grams

BREAKFAST— 20 grams	LUNCH— 11 grams	DINNER— 28 grams
½ cup fresh straw-berries, sour cream 2 slices grilled ham 1 thin slice buttered protein toast	Eggs in aspic Endive salad 1 soda cracker with cream cheese	Pork chops Sauerkraut in white wine 1 small boiled potato Baked custard

TOTAL FOR THE DAY: 59 grams

BREAKFAST— 21 grams	LUNCH— 14 grams	DINNER— 22 grams
½ cup grapefruit juice 2 scrambled eggs 1 thin slice buttered rye toast	Veal scallopini Asparagus with Hollandaise sauce ½ fresh apple with cheese	Brandywine beef Turkish eggplant Coffee fluff

TOTAL FOR THE DAY: 57 grams

BREAKFAST— 12 grams	LUNCH— 24 grams	DINNER— 24 grams
2 fried eggs and bacon 1 thin slice buttered toast	1 cup oyster stew 1 soda cracker Fresh peach	Beef stew (without potatoes) Raw mushroom salad Gelatin dessert with whipped cream

TOTAL FOR THE DAY: 60 grams

BREAKFAST— 25 grams	LUNCH— 21 grams	DINNER— 12 grams
½ cup orange juice 2 baked eggs 1 thin slice buttered toast	Broiled salmon Raw cauliflowerets vinaigrette ½ cup ice cream with 1 tsp. pistachio nuts	Roast beef Green beans with almond butter 1 dessert American pancake spread with gingered cream cheese

TOTAL FOR THE DAY: 58 grams

BREAKFAST— 18 grams	LUNCH— 12·5 grams	DINNER— 23·5 grams
½ tangerine 1 poached egg on 1 thin slice buttered toast	Shrimp salad in half tomato 2 soda crackers with cream cheese	Roast chicken Boiled globe artichoke, lemon butter Celery sticks 1 thin slice sponge cake

TOTAL FOR THE DAY: 54 grams

BREAKFAST— 22 grams	LUNCH— 18 grams	DINNER— 14 grams
½ cup tomato juice Puffy Omelette Chasseur 1 thin slice buttered toast	Steamed trout with lemon ½ cup green peas 1 small tangerine	Burgundy baked chicken Cabbage served with butter Green salad with red onion rings Slice of cheese

TOTAL FOR THE DAY: 54 grams

BREAKFAST— 28 grams	LUNCH— 19 grams	DINNER— 13 grams
½ cup grapefruit juice 2 American pancakes with 1 tsp. syrup	Chicken broth with celery 1 soda cracker Egg salad ½ cup blueberries with cream	Lemon veal with olives Green salad with Roquefort dressing Baked custard made with artificial sweetener

TOTAL FOR THE DAY: 60 grams

BREAKFAST— 18 grams	LUNCH— 24 grams	DINNER— 17 grams
½ cup tomato juice 2 fried eggs with ham 1 thin slice buttered toast	Beef bouillon with sliced mushrooms and chives 1 thin slice bread spread with cream cheese Slice of honeydew melon	2 chopped sirloin patties Cauliflower with Hollandaise sauce 1 thin slice sponge cake with dollop of whipped cream

TOTAL FOR THE DAY: 59 grams

LOW CARBOHYDRATE RECIPES

BAKED EGGS WITH ANCHOVY

1 *can anchovies*
1 *cup heavy cream*
¼ *lb. mushrooms, sliced*
1 *tbs. butter*
2 *tbs. chopped parsley*
Freshly ground pepper
4 *eggs*
¼ *cup grated Parmesan cheese*

Preheat oven to 400 degrees F.

1. Mash anchovies in bottom of a 4-cup baking dish. Add cream and mix well. Bake until mixture begins to bubble.
2. Sauté mushrooms in butter until soft. Add to cream, and add parsley. Continue baking until mixture is reduced by about a third. Season to taste with pepper. Turn off oven heat.
3. Remove baking dish from oven, but leave oven door closed to retain heat. Break each egg into a saucer and slide carefully into sauce. Sprinkle with grated cheese. Return to lowest part of oven, and cook gently until eggs are set.

BRANDYWINE BEEF

3 *lb. boneless chuck or other beef suitable for potting*
⅛ *tsp. cinnamon*
Freshly ground pepper
Salt
2 *tbs. cooking oil*
1 *small onion, sliced*
1 *clove garlic (optional)*
1 *bay leaf*
3 *tbs. brandy (or bourbon)*
½ *cup dry white wine*

1. Sprinkle meat with salt, pepper, and cinnamon. Be meagre with cinnamon!
2. Heat oil in a large pot over a medium high heat, until hot but not smoking. Add meat and brown it well on all sides.
3. Add the onion slices and let them brown. Add garlic if desired.

4. Reduce heat. Heat brandy, ignite, and pour over meat. Spoon the burning brandy over the meat until the flame dies.
5. Add the bay leaf and wine, cover tightly, reduce heat, and cook about 1½ hours, or until meat is fork tender but not too soft. It should retain a little firmness. After first hour of cooking, turn the meat over and taste gravy to adjust seasonings.
6. When meat is done, remove it to a hot platter. Remove bay leaf, increase heat under liquid and boil rapidly until reduced by a third. To serve, cut meat into ½-inch slices and pour gravy over it.

CHICKEN WITH CURRY CREAM

1 *roasting chicken (2½ to 3 lb.) cut into quarters*
5 *tbs. butter*
1 *onion, sliced*
¼ *cup chicken broth*
Salt and pepper to taste
¼ *cup cognac or bourbon*
½ *tsp. curry powder*
1 *cup heavy cream*
1 *tbs. chopped parsley*

1. In a heavy skillet, brown the chicken pieces lightly on both sides, using 3 tbs. butter. Transfer to a small Dutch oven containing the remaining two tbs. of butter. Sprinkle onion slices over the chicken.
2. Pour chicken broth into the skillet, scrape up browned particles and pour all over chicken. Sprinkle with salt and pepper. Cover tightly, and simmer slowly until chicken is tender (about 45 minutes or longer).
3. Pour off liquid into a small saucepan, and boil rapidly until reduced to about one-third of original quantity. Meanwhile, pour cognac over chicken and cook gently while completing sauce.
4. Mix curry powder with 2 tbs. heavy cream. Pour over chicken. Add remaining cream to reduced liquid in saucepan, and heat but do not boil. Pour over chicken. Sprinkle with chopped parsley.

CHILE RELLENOS
(Stuffed Chillies with Cheese)

8 *green chillies or Italian peppers*
½ *lb. Monterey Jack cheese or sharp Cheddar sliced into 8 fingers*
4 *eggs, separated*
¼ *tsp. salt*
Oil for deep frying

1. Char the skins of the peppers by holding each on a fork over a gas flame. When chilli is black all over, roll in a wet paper towel. When all are charred, rub skins off with a dry cloth. Slit each pepper down one side, open it flat and remove *all* the seeds and the core.
2. Place a finger of cheese in the centre of each chilli, and close the chilli over it. Chill until ready to use.
3. In a mixing bowl beat 4 egg yolks until they are very stiff and pale yellow. Add ⅛ tsp. salt.
4. In another bowl, beat egg whites with ⅛ tsp. salt until they are quite stiff. Fold the whites thoroughly into the yolks.
5. Fill a large heavy skillet to a depth of 2 inches with oil, and heat to a moderate frying temperature.
6. Dip chillies, one at a time, into eggs. With a large spoon, remove each chilli, taking with it as much egg as spoon will hold, and slide it into the hot fat. Cook until one side is light brown, then turn and cook until other side is brown. Drain on absorbent paper and arrange in a baking dish. Keep warm. Serve with following Mexican Sauce.

MEXICAN SAUCE

2 tbs. butter
1 clove garlic, chopped
1 small onion, chopped
1 cup tomato purée, or 1 medium can tomatoes
1 tsp. chilli powder
¼ tsp. salt

1. Melt butter, add garlic and onion. Cook until onion is soft.
2. Add tomato purée, chilli powder, and salt. Cook for 5 minutes. If canned tomatoes are used, mash the tomatoes while cooking until mixture has reduced and thickened. Pour sauce over chillies.

CHICKEN WITH FENNEL

1 3-lb. broiling chicken cut into serving pieces
¼ cup butter
½ tsp. salt
⅛ tsp. freshly ground black pepper
¼ lb. fresh mushrooms, sliced
1 tbs. fennel seeds
1 tbs. chopped chives or green onion
1½ cups sour cream
1 tbs. lemon juice
1 tsp. grated lemon rind
1 tbs. chopped parsley

Preheat oven to 325 degrees F.

1. Melt butter in a large skillet and brown chicken well on all sides. Transfer chicken to a casserole.
2. Add salt, pepper, mushrooms, fennel seeds, and chives to pan drippings, and cook, stirring until mushrooms are soft and done. Add sour cream, stir and cook gently until sour cream is heated through. Pour sauce over chicken.
3. Cover and bake 25–30 minutes, or until chicken is tender. Stir in lemon juice and rind. Sprinkle with parsley.

FEGATO AGRODOLCE
(Sweet and Sour Liver)

1½ lb. calf's liver, cut into 1" strips
2 tbs. butter
2 tbs. olive oil
1 medium onion, thinly sliced
1 tbs. pine nuts
2 tbs. wine vinegar
3 tbs. chicken broth
Artificial sweetener equal to 2 tsp. sugar
½ tsp. grated bitter chocolate
Pinch of salt
Dash of cayenne pepper
1 tbs. butter

1. In a saucepan, heat butter and oil together. Add onions and pine nuts and sauté until onions are soft and golden.
2. Add wine vinegar, chicken broth, sweetener, and grated chocolate. Stir over low heat for 5 minutes. Season.
3. In a frying pan, heat 1 tbs. butter. Add liver and sauté quickly over high heat just until done.
4. Lower heat, pour sauce over liver and cook for one minute or until heated.

EGGS IN ASPIC

4 eggs, poached and cooled (reserve and crush 2 shells)
4 cups strong chicken broth, room temperature
⅛ tsp. dried tarragon leaves
2 tsp. lemon juice
2 tbs. dry vermouth
1 egg white
2 envelopes unflavoured gelatin
4 stuffed olives for decoration
6 thin slices ham, cut into ovals

1. Add tarragon, lemon juice, and wine to chicken broth. Beat in egg white and crushed egg shells. Bring to a boil, and strain through a clean, wet, finely woven cotton cloth or several layers of cheese-cloth which have been rinsed in hot water.

2. Remove ½ cup broth, cool quickly. Dissolve gelatin in it.
3. Stir remaining hot broth into gelatin mixture. Heat until gelatin is completely dissolved. Chill until syrupy but still liquid.
4. Slice olives. Spoon a thin layer of gelatin mixture into bottom of four 1-cup moulds. Chill until firm. Arrange stuffed olive slices into desired pattern, and cover with another layer of gelatin mixture. Chill until firm.
5. Trim poached eggs with round pastry cutter or paring knife. Place one egg in each mould, and cover with layer of chilled, syrupy gelatin mixture, until not quite full. Place a slice of ham on each mould, and cover with a layer of remaining aspic. Chill several hours, or until quite firm.
6. Unmould on to serving dish. Garnish as desired (watercress, capers, and/or mayonnaise go well atop these).

HAMBURGERS WITH BORDELAISE SAUCE

1 tbs. butter
¼ cup minced onion
1 lb. minced beef
1 egg, lightly beaten
1 tsp. salt
⅛ tsp. pepper
⅛ tsp. poultry seasoning

1. Melt butter in a small saucepan. Add chopped onion and sauté until soft and golden. Cool.
2. Add cooked onion and all remaining ingredients to hamburger, and beat well. Form into four patties.
3. Pan-fry hamburgers in a heavy skillet, using 1 tbs. butter and 1 tbs. oil, to desired doneness, preferably rare. To serve, spoon Bordelaise sauce over patties.

BORDELAISE SAUCE

(Can be prepared in advance)

1 tbs. butter
1 strip bacon, diced
½ carrot, thinly sliced
3 tbs. chopped onion
1 sprig parsley
½ bay leaf
Pinch of thyme
1 small soda cracker, finely crushed
1½ cups consommé, heated
1 tsp. tomato paste
¼ cup diced beef marrow (optional)
2 tsp. chopped green onion
½ cup claret or dry red wine
Pepper
½ tsp. lemon juice
½ tbs. sweet butter

1. In a heavy skillet, heat 1 tbs. butter with diced bacon. Cook until bacon is crisp.
2. Add sliced carrot, onion, parsley, bay leaf, thyme. Cook, stirring, until onion is golden. Add crushed soda cracker. Stir until lightly browned. Slowly add hot consommé and tomato paste. Cover, simmer until vegetables are very soft, about 20 to 30 minutes. Uncover, increase heat slightly, and simmer until reduced to ⅔ cup. Strain. If beef marrow is used, add to sauce, simmer 4 minutes, strain again and reserve marrow.
3. In same skillet, mix chopped green onion, wine, dash of pepper. Simmer ten minutes, until wine is reduced to one tablespoon. Add strained sauce, simmer until reduced to ½ cup. Strain. Add poached marrow, lemon juice and ½ tsp. butter.

Note: Bordelaise sauce is also good with rare steak, roast beef, filet mignon.

LEMON VEAL WITH OLIVES

3 *lb. boneless veal, rolled and tied*
2 *tbs. grated lemon rind (use fresh lemon rind)*
1 *clove garlic, finely minced*
¾ *tsp. salt*
¼ *tsp. pepper*
½ *tsp. dried rosemary leaves, crushed*
¼ *tsp. dried sweet basil leaves, crushed*
3 *tbs. olive oil*
½ *cup dry Marsala wine*
½ *cup pitted ripe olives, sliced*

1. Mix lemon rind, garlic, salt, pepper, rosemary, and basil. Divide this mixture in half. Untie and unroll the veal and rub the inner surface with one-half of the flavouring mixture. Reroll and retie. Rub the remaining mixture all over the outside of the veal.
2. Heat the olive oil over a medium high flame in a heavy pot large enough to hold the veal. Brown the veal lightly.
3. Pour the wine over the veal, reduce the heat to low, cover tightly and simmer about 1½ hours, or until veal is fork tender, but not too soft. Turn the veal occasionally. Be careful not to overcook.
4. When done, remove the veal to a hot platter and let it stand. There should be quite a bit of liquid in the pan.

Increase the heat and boil until liquid is reduced to about half. Add the sliced ripe olives and heat through. The sauce should thicken somewhat on being reduced.
5. Slice the veal and spoon the sauce over it.

NING PO SPINACH

2 lb. spinach cleaned, drained
3 qt. boiling water
2 tbs. oil
3 cloves garlic, chopped
1 tsp. salt
Artificial sweetener equal to 2 tsp. sugar

1. Plunge spinach into boiling water. Boil 1 minute and drain.
2. Heat oil in a large skillet, add garlic and cook until lightly browned. Add spinach, stir rapidly over high heat for three or four minutes.
3. Sprinkle with salt and sweetener. Mix well and serve hot or cold.

Note: This makes a good filling for a luncheon or light supper omelette.

LAMB SHANKS BRAZIL

4 lamb shanks
1 tbs. olive oil
½ tsp. salt
Freshly ground pepper
2 thin slices of lemon
1 clove of garlic
1 bay leaf
½ cup strong coffee (more if required)

1. Heat oil over moderately high heat in a large Dutch oven or heavy pot with a tight lid. Lightly brown lamb shanks, sprinkle with salt and pepper. Add lemon, garlic, bay leaf, and coffee. Heat until liquid boils.
2. Cover pot tightly, reduce heat to very low, and simmer meat slowly for 1 hour. Check seasonings and add more coffee if necessary. Continue cooking another ½ hour, until meat is very tender.
3. Remove meat to a warm platter. Increase heat under liquid and boil rapidly until reduced by about one-third. Pour over shanks.

LAMB WITH RADISH SAUCE

4 generous slices of cold roast lamb
20 small red radishes, as nearly uniform as possible
1 cup chicken broth
2 tbs. sweet butter
1 small unsalted soda cracker, finely crushed
1 heaping tsp. prepared horse-radish sauce

Preheat oven to 350 degrees F.

1. Arrange lamb slices in a low oven-proof casserole.
2. Cook radishes in the chicken broth for 8–10 minutes, or until they are barely beginning to soften. The broth will turn a pale pink.
3. Remove radishes from broth, and arrange them over the lamb.
4. In a small saucepan, melt the butter, add the crushed soda cracker and stir until mixed. Slowly add the hot chicken broth and stir until smooth and slightly thick. Stir in horseradish sauce. Pour over the lamb.
5. Heat the dish in preheated oven until meat is heated and sauce is bubbly.

MOCK BOAR (Marinated Pork)

3 lb. boneless pork roast

Seasonings:

½ tsp. freshly ground black pepper
1 tsp. salt
¼ tsp. allspice
1 bay leaf, crumbled
¼ tsp. caraway seed, crushed
⅛ tsp. celery seed
¼ tsp. thyme
¼ tsp. tarragon
¼ tsp. sage
4 coriander seeds
4 juniper berries
⅛ tsp. cinnamon
½ tsp. grated orange rind

Mix the above ingredients and rub well into pork. Place pork in a large bowl.

Marinade:

1 small onion, chopped
1 small carrot, chopped
1 clove garlic, halved
¼ cup olive oil
1 cup dry red wine
¼ cup wine vinegar
1 tbs. cognac

Slowly sauté onion, carrot, and garlic in oil. Add wine and vinegar and bring to a boil, add cognac and pour over pork. Cover, refrigerate, and let pork stand in marinade from 24 hours to 3 days. Turn and baste several times a day.

To Cook:

Marinated pork
2 *tbs. cooking oil*
1 *small onion, sliced*
1 *small carrot, sliced*
Medium herb bouquet: 4 *parsley sprigs,* ½ *bay leaf,* ¼ *tsp. thyme tied in cheesecloth*
¼ *cup dry vermouth or canned bouillon*

Preheat oven to 325 degrees F.

1. Remove pork from marinade. Drain for ½ hour. Dry thoroughly with paper towels, scraping off all marinade.
2. Heat oil in large casserole over moderately high heat. Add pork and brown on all sides. Remove to a warm dish.
3. Pour all but 2 tablespoons of fat from casserole. Stir in vegetables. Cook slowly for 5 minutes. Add herb bouquet.
4. Return meat to casserole, insert meat thermometer, and cover. Roast for about 2 hours or until thermometer reads 180 degrees. Baste roast two or three times during cooking period. Pork should cook slowly and evenly, so that it will render juices.
5. When pork is done, remove to a hot serving platter. Remove any trussing strings.
6. Pour wine into the casserole, and simmer for 2 or 3 minutes. Remove herb bouquet and as much fat as possible from surface of liquid, and mash the vegetables. Cook gravy rapidly until reduced to about one cup. Pour into a hot gravy boat and serve separately with pork.

ROAST DUCKLING WITH GIBLET SAUCE

2 *small ducklings, about* 4 *lb. each*
Salt, pepper, thyme
2 *small onions, sliced*
3 *small carrots*
2 *small onions, coarsely chopped*
1½ *cups beef bouillon*
Duck gizzard, heart, and neck cut into 1*-inch pieces. Reserve liver for later cooking*
2 *tbs. oil*
Herb bouquet: 2 *parsley sprigs, small bay leaf,* ¼ *tsp. sage*
¼ *cup port wine or burgundy*

Preheat oven to 425 degrees F.

1. Season duck cavities with salt, pepper, and a pinch of thyme. Stuff each with a small sliced onion. Tie legs, wings, and neck skin tightly to body and place breast up in a shallow roasting pan. Slice two of the carrots and one onion and sprinkle around the birds. Cook until lightly browned, about 15 minutes.
2. Reduce oven to 350 degrees F., turn ducks breast down, and roast for 30 minutes. Take care that fat does not burn. Turn ducks breast up and cook until duck is done, about 30 minutes. (*Note:* Duck is medium rare if juices from thigh run pale rosy when meat is pricked. Duck is well done when juices run pale yellow.)
3. While duck is roasting, prepare stock for sauce. Brown cut up giblets, 1 carrot cut up, and 1 onion chopped in hot oil. Add bouillon and the herb bouquet. Simmer until giblets are very tender, about 1 hour, adding water if necessary.
4. When duck is done, drain cavity juices into stock, and place duck on a warm platter. Set in a turned-off oven with door left ajar while preparing sauce.
5. Pour juices remaining in roasting pan into a bowl, and remove as much fat as possible. Add these juices to stock. Remove herb bouquet from stock, then pour stock back into roasting pan, place over high heat, and cook, stirring and scraping browned particles from bottom of pan. Crush the vegetables. Add wine and cut up liver, and cook until liver is just done. Correct seasonings. Serve over duck.

PARMA VEAL

2 *lb. scallopini of veal, pounded*
½ *cup grated Parmesan cheese*
4 *tbs. butter*
1 *cup fresh mushroom caps, sliced*
Salt, dash cayenne pepper
1 *tsp. meat extract dissolved into 3 tbs. beef stock*
¼ *cup dry wine*

1. Coat scallopini on both sides with grated cheese.
2. Heat 2 tbs. butter in frying pan. Brown veal on both sides.
3. In a separate pan, sauté sliced mushrooms in remaining butter. Season lightly with salt and cayenne pepper.
4. Add meat extract and stock. Simmer for 2 minutes.
5. Add wine, bring to a boil, and pour over scallopini. Simmer 2 minutes.

ORIENT BEEF

1½ lb. sirloin tip, thinly sliced
Small piece beef suet
½ cup condensed consommé
⅓ cup soy sauce
1 small head Chinese cabbage sliced crosswise
½ lb. mushrooms, sliced
¼ cup canned bamboo shoots, sliced
12 green onions, thinly sliced
1 bunch watercress
½ lb. spinach washed, drained

1. Heat a large skillet, and rub with a cube of beet suet. Add consommé and soy sauce, sliced Chinese cabbage, mushrooms, bamboo shoots, and green onions. Cook for 5 minutes over high heat, stirring.
2. Add meat, watercress, and spinach. Cook, stirring, for 5 minutes longer, or until ingredients are cooked, but vegetables are still crisp.

GARLIC CHICKEN

2 whole heads of garlic (35 to 40 cloves), broken into cloves
¼ cup olive oil
4 stalks celery, cut into thin strips
6 sprigs parsley
1 tbs. tarragon
1 small roasting chicken or capon, cut into 8 serving pieces, or 8 leg and thigh pieces
Salt
Freshly ground black pepper
Nutmeg
⅓ cup cognac (or brandy or bourbon)
¼ tsp. salt
Pastry seal: ¾ cup flour mixed with enough water to form a thick paste

Preheat oven to moderately high 375 degrees F.

1. Drop garlic cloves into boiling water, boil two minutes, drain, and peel. Reserve.
2. Pour oil into a large casserole. Add celery, parsley, and tarragon. Toss to mix and coat with oil.
3. Sprinkle chicken pieces lightly with salt, pepper, and nutmeg. Add to oil and vegetable mixture, and turn to coat each piece thoroughly.
4. Sprinkle with garlic cloves. Add cognac and ¼ tsp. salt.
5. Cover casserole with lid. Spread pastry seal (flour and water paste) around seam between lid and casserole to seal them together. Completely cover top and seal with aluminium foil.

6. Bake casserole for 1½ hours. Do not remove foil seal or lid until ready to serve. The chicken may be served directly from the casserole. Otherwise, remove it to a hot platter. Put the sauce through a purèer or a blender, reheat, and pour over chicken.

Note: Don't worry about the amount of garlic used. Because it is not crushed or chopped, the sauce is not overpowering, but has a rich, distinctive flavour.

PORK CHOPS CHARCUTIÈRE

4 lean pork chops, 1 *inch thick*
Salt and freshly ground black pepper to taste
1 *tbs. vegetable oil*
4 *tbs. shallots or green onion tops*
1 *tbs. finely chopped onion*
1 *small soda cracker, very finely crushed*
½ *cup dry white wine or dry vermouth*
1 *cup beef bouillon, consommé, or stock*
1 *tbs. Dijon-style mustard*
2 *tbs. sweet butter*
3 *small gherkins, cut into strips*

1. Trim pork chops, leaving just a thin layer of fat. Sprinkle lightly with salt and pepper.
2. Heat oil in a large skillet and brown chops on both sides. Cook until done (about 30 minutes). Slit near bone to be sure chops are done through. Transfer to warm platter; cover to keep warm.
3. Add shallots and onion to skillet, cook, stirring, for 2 minutes. Stir in crushed soda cracker.
4. Slowly add wine, stir to dissolve brown particles in pan. Cook rapidly, stirring until wine is reduced to ¼ cup. Reduce heat, slowly add hot bouillon. Cook, stirring, for 10 minutes.
5. Mix mustard and butter together. Swirl into sauce. Add gherkins. Add chops and heat through. To serve, spoon some sauce over each chop, and serve remaining sauce from a sauceboat.

STUFFED CHICKEN BREASTS, KIEV STYLE

4 *half breasts of chicken, skin left on and main wing bones left attached*
1 *small onion, finely chopped*
2 *tbs. butter for sautéing*
¼ *lb. chicken livers, cut in half*

¼ lb. mushrooms, coarsely chopped
Salt and freshly ground black pepper
1 tbs. parsley, finely chopped
2 tbs. soft butter
Fat for deep frying

1. In a medium skillet, sauté onion in 1 tbs. of butter until transparent. Remove, leaving as much butter as possible in skillet.
2. Add 1 tbs. butter and chicken livers and sauté livers just until done. They should be slightly rare. Remove and add to onions.
3. Add mushrooms to skillet, and sauté until soft. Add, together with whatever butter remains in pan, to onion and liver mixture.
4. Grind onion, liver, and mushrooms with medium blade of grinder, or chop with a chopper until fairly fine. Season to taste with salt and pepper, add parsley, and blend with 2 tbs. soft butter. Chill until firm.
5. Place each breast between two sheets of waxed paper and pound thin with a wooden mallet. Do not split flesh.
6. Form liver mixture into finger-shaped pieces. Place a piece in middle of each breast, roll up, letting wing bone protrude, and making sides overlap. Use skin to enclose flesh, and secure with toothpick or tie with fine string.
7. Fill a frying pan with enough oil to cover breasts completely. Heat to 360 degrees F. Fry chicken until a deep, golden brown. Drain on absorbent paper. Before, serving, place paper frill on wing bone.

SAUERKRAUT IN WHITE WINE

1 small onion, minced
2 tbs. butter
1 qt. sauerkraut, drained (canned or bulk)
1 small tart apple, chopped
1 tsp. caraway seed
1 cup chicken stock
1 cup dry white wine

1. Sauté onion in butter until pale brown.
2. Add to sauerkraut with apple and caraway seed, and turn into a greased casserole. Add stock and white wine.
3. Bake, covered, in a medium oven (350 degrees F.) for 45 minutes to 1½ hours. Use shorter time for canned kraut, longer time for bulk kraut.

Note: If kraut seems excessively salty before cooking, rinse with cold water. This method of preparing kraut makes it particularly suited to serving with pork, roast duck or goose, or grilled pork chops.

CHICKEN BREASTS À LA SUISSE

4 *whole chicken breasts boned, skinned, and pounded to ¼ inch thick*
4 *thin slices baked or boiled ham*
1 *pimento, cut in strips*
4 *thin slices Swiss cheese*
¼ *cup butter*
1 *cup dry white wine*
⅛ *tsp. nutmeg*
Salt and pepper to taste
1 *tbs. onion, finely chopped*
1 *cup sour cream*
2 *egg yolks, lightly beaten*

1. Place a slice of ham, a strip of pimento, and a slice of cheese on one side of each breast. Fold second side over to cover filling. Secure with a toothpick.
2. Heat butter in a frying pan over medium high heat. When butter is hot but not smoking, sauté breasts on all sides until golden. Lower heat, add ¾ cup of the wine, the nutmeg, salt, and pepper to taste. Cover, cook slowly until chicken is tender, about 15 minutes.
3. Remove chicken to a warm platter; keep warm. Add onion to the pan. Cook three minutes. Stir in remaining wine. Mix sour cream with egg yolks, and stir slowly into sauce. Heat, stirring until thickened. Do not allow to boil. Check seasonings. Pour into sauce boat, and serve separately to pour over breasts.

Note: Dry Vermouth may be substituted for the dry white wine in this recipe. If you wish, omit the ham—you'll hardly miss it—but never the cheese.

PUFFY OMELETTE CHASSEUR

4 *tbs. butter*
2 *tsp. chopped shallots*
3 *chicken livers cut into four pieces each*
4 *medium mushrooms, coarsely chopped*
Salt and pepper
3 *tbs. white wine or chicken stock*
8 *eggs*
⅛ *tsp. salt*
1 *cup milk*
12 *small mushroom caps, sautéed*
1 *tsp. chopped parsley*

1. In a medium skillet, melt 2 tbs. butter and add shallots. Cook, stirring, for 1 minute, or until soft. Add chicken livers and mushrooms, sprinkle with salt and pepper. Cook gently until liver is just done. Do not overcook.
2. Add dry white wine or stock, and cook, stirring, for 2 or 3 minutes. Use as filling for omelette.
3. Break eggs into a large bowl. Add $\frac{1}{8}$ tsp. salt and beat with a large wire whisk or electric beater until very frothy. Add milk and beat again until frothy.
4. Melt 2 tbs. of butter in a very large skillet over high heat. When butter is hot, but not smoking, pour in omelette mixture. Cover, keep on high heat for 15 seconds, then quickly reduce heat to very low and cook for 8–10 minutes. Peek under lid. Eggs should have puffed up and have a smooth, satiny look. If they haven't puffed up, continue cooking.
5. When eggs are done, spread Chasseur Sauce over one-half. Using a large spatula, carefully fold other half over sauce. Turn omelette out on to a large, warm platter. Garnish with sautéed mushroom caps and sprinkle with chopped parsley.

TURKISH EGGPLANT

1 *small head of garlic (8 or 10 cloves)*
2 *medium eggplants, sliced (it is not necessary to peel them)*
2 *medium onions, chopped*
3 *cups chopped green pepper*
6 *sliced tomatoes, or 1 can of tomatoes*
Salt
$\frac{1}{2}$ *cup olive oil*

Preheat oven to 300 degrees F.

1. Blanch garlic cloves by placing in boiling water and boiling for 2 minutes. Peel and chop.
2. Lightly oil a large, heavy casserole. Cover the bottom with a solid layer of eggplant slices. Sprinkle some of the garlic over it. Add a layer of chopped onion, then green pepper, and then tomato. Sprinkle lightly with salt. Repeat until all vegetables are used.
3. If canned tomatoes are used, pour juice from can over mixture, and finally sprinkle olive oil over the top.
4. Bake at 300 degrees F. for 3 hours or 250 degrees F. for 5 hours. This dish should have a custardy texture.

GREEN BEANS WITH BROWN BUTTER GARLIC SAUCE

1 lb. green beans
3 quarts boiling water
4½ tsp. salt
¼ cup butter
1 clove garlic, thinly sliced
¼ cup chopped onion
¼ tsp. salt

1. Trim ends off washed and drained green beans. Cut in half or into 2-inch lengths.
2. Add 4½ tsp. salt to the 3 quarts of boiling water. Slip beans by handfuls into water, making sure water continues to boil rapidly. Lower heat, leave uncovered and simmer for 6–8 minutes. Beans should be done, but crisp, with bright green colour. Drain at once. If they are not to be used immediately, run cold water over them, drain, and dry in paper towels. Place in a covered bowl until ready to use.
3. Melt butter in a small saucepan over low heat. When it begins to darken and turn pale brown, add sliced garlic. Butter will foam up. Remove from heat until foam subsides. Garlic should be pale brown around the edges. Add chopped onion and cook until onion is soft. Add salt.
4. Pour butter mixture into a large frying pan. Add green beans and toss or stir with a wooden spoon over low flame until beans are heated through.

VEAL KIDNEYS WITH MUSTARD SAUCE

4 veal kidneys, whole, but fat and filament removed
4 tbs. butter
2 tbs. minced shallots or green onion
½ cup dry vermouth
1 tbs. lemon juice
1½ tbs. Dijon-style mustard
2 tbs. soft butter
Salt and pepper
3 tbs. chopped parsley or chives

1. Heat butter in a shallow casserole or chafing dish. When foam subsides, roll kidneys in butter. Cook, uncovered, for about 10 minutes, over medium heat, turning every 2 minutes. When kidneys are light brown, firm, and slightly puffy, remove to a hot plate, cover, and keep warm.
2. Add shallots to butter in casserole, and cook for 1 or 2 minutes. Add wine and lemon juice, and boil, stirring and

scraping up browned particles, until wine is reduced by half.

3. Mix mustard and two tbs. butter, and swirl into wine. Add salt and pepper to taste.

4. Cut kidneys crosswise into ¼-inch slices. Sprinkle lightly with salt and pepper. Return kidneys to casserole. Stir over low heat only long enough to warm through. Do not allow sauce to boil. Sprinkle with chopped parsley or chives.

BURGUNDY BAKED CHICKEN

1 broiling chicken, cut into 8 pieces
½ cup mild oil, preferably peanut oil (not olive oil)
1 medium onion, coarsely chopped
2 cloves garlic, minced
¼ tsp. oregano
½ tsp. salt
2 tbs. lemon juice
1 cup Burgundy wine, or other good, dry red wine

Preheat oven to 350 degrees F.

1. Pour oil into a large skillet and heat over high heat until very hot, almost smoking. Add chicken pieces and sauté until a rich, golden brown. Remove chicken, drain on paper towels and place in a small, covered roasting pan.

2. Remove all except 2 tbs. of oil from the frying pan. Lower heat, add onion, garlic, oregano, salt, and lemon juice. Simmer over low heat until onion is soft and yellow, about 5 minutes.

3. Sprinkle onion mixture over chicken. Cover and bake ½ hour. Correct seasoning.

4. Bring wine to a boil and pour over chicken. Cook, uncovered, for 10 more minutes.

FILLED DESSERT CRÊPES

¾ cup sifted flour
⅛ tsp. salt
3 eggs
Liquid sweetener equal to 2 tbs. sugar
2 scant tbs. brandy
2 scant tbs. melted butter
½–⅔ cup milk
Sweet butter for frying
Filling: 1 scant tsp. jam or 1 tbs. sliced fresh strawberries for each crêpe

1. Sift flour with salt.

2 Beat in eggs one at a time.

3. Add sweetener and beat batter until smooth.
4. Mix in brandy and butter. Mix in milk until batter has the consistency of light cream.
5. Set aside in cool place for at least 1 hour, longer if possible. Beat again before using.
6. Melt about 1 tsp. sweet butter in small skillet. Over medium heat spoon in just enough batter to cover bottom. As edges of crêpe turn brown, run a spatula around to loosen them. Crêpe is ready to be turned when top is dry. Turn with spatula and brown the other side.
7. Spread each crêpe with jam or fill with 1 tbs. sliced strawberries and roll or fold.

Note: This recipe may seem wildly extravagant in carbohydrates, but it makes 12 thin crêpes. Total carbohydrate content of each thus comes to less than 5 grams per crêpe, plus 10 more grams if you splurge on jam or approximately 15 grams for sliced strawberries. The other 11 crêpes will have to go to the non-dieters—but isn't one better than none?

COFFEE FLUFF

6 *egg yolks*
Liquid sweetener equal to 5 *tsp. sugar*
Few grains of salt
¾ *cup strong coffee*

1. Combine egg yolks, liquid sweetener, and salt in the top of a double boiler. Beat with a rotary beater—electric or hand—until the mixture is very thick.
2. Place over simmering water—do not let the water boil—and gradually add the coffee as you continue to beat. Beat until the pudding thickens and forms a mound when dropped from the beater.
3. Chill, covered, until ready to serve.

LEMON CHIFFON PUDDING

1 *tbs. unflavoured gelatin*
¼ *cup water*
½ *cup lemon juice*
½ *tsp. salt*
4 *egg yolks, well beaten*
Liquid sweetener to equal ½ *cup sugar*
1 *tsp. grated lemon rind*
4 *egg whites*
1 *cup heavy cream*

1. Soak gelatin in water.
2. In top of double boiler, combine lemon juice, salt, egg yolks. Water in bottom of double boiler should not touch top. Cook, stirring, until mixture begins to thicken. Add sweetener and continue cooking until mixture is very thick.
3. Stir in gelatin and grated rind.
4. When mixture has cooled, beat egg whites until stiff. Beat lemon mixture and fold in egg whites.
5. Beat cream until stiff. Fold into lemon mixture. Spoon into 6 small sherbet glasses or custard cups and chill several hours before serving.

Note: This recipe will make 6 small (carbohydrates: 4 grams) or 4 lavish (carbohydrates: 6 grams) servings. Let your arithmetic be your guide.

CUSTARD CRÈME

2 cups heavy cream
4 egg yolks
Liquid sweetener eq. to 3 tbs. sugar
⅛ tsp. salt
1 tsp. vanilla extract

1. In the top of a double boiler, scald cream.
2. Beat egg yolks well. Add sweetener, salt, and mix well.
3. Pour a small amount of the scalded cream into the egg yolks and blend well.
4. Pour egg-cream mixture into the remaining cream and cook, stirring constantly, until the mixture is thickened and coats the spoon—a matter of 4 minutes or less. Stir in vanilla extract.
5. Pour into individual serving dishes. Chill thoroughly.